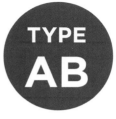

TYPE
AB

Eat Right 4 Your Type

PERSONALIZED COOKBOOK

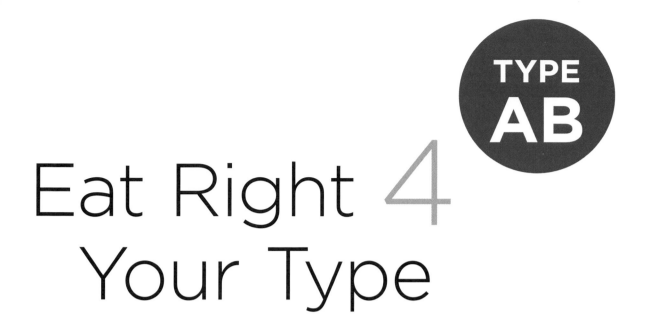

TYPE AB

Eat Right 4 Your Type

PERSONALIZED COOKBOOK

**150+ Healthy Recipes
For Your Blood Type Diet®**

Dr. Peter J. D'Adamo
with Kristin O'Connor

Photographs by Kristin O'Connor

Previously published as *Personalized Living
Using the Blood Type Diet® (Type AB)*

BERKLEY BOOKS, NEW YORK

THE BERKLEY PUBLISHING GROUP
Published by the Penguin Group
Penguin Group (USA) LLC
375 Hudson Street, New York, New York 10014, USA

USA | Canada | UK | Ireland | Australia | New Zealand | India | South Africa | China

Penguin Books Ltd., Registered Offices: 80 Strand, London WC2R 0RL, England
For more information about the Penguin Group, visit penguin.com.

Library of Congress Cataloging-in-Publication Data

D'Adamo, Peter J.
  Eat right 4 your type personalized cookbook type AB : 150+ healthy recipes for your blood
type diet / Dr. Peter J. D'Adamo with Kristin O'Connor ; photographs by Kristin O'Connor.
    p. cm.
  ISBN 978-0-425-26946-6 (pbk.)
  1. Diet therapy. 2. Nutrition. 3. Blood groups. 4. Naturopathy. I. O'Connor, Kristin. II.
Title. III. Title: Eat right for your type personalized cookbook type AB.
  RM219.D289 2013
  641.5'631—dc23
                            2013021044

PUBLISHING HISTORY
Previously published in eBook format as *Personalized Living Using the Blood Type Diet®*
(Type AB) by Drum Hill Publishing LLC in 2012
Berkley trade paperback edition / October 2013

PRINTED IN THE UNITED STATES OF AMERICA

10   9   8   7   6   5   4   3

Cover design by Jason Gill
Cover photo by Christopher Bierlein
Book design by Pauline Neuwirth

ALWAYS LEARNING   PEARSON

Contents

Type AB ⬤ v

Lunch

Dinner

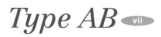

Type AB vii

Snacks

Drinks and Beverages

Type AB

Type AB xi

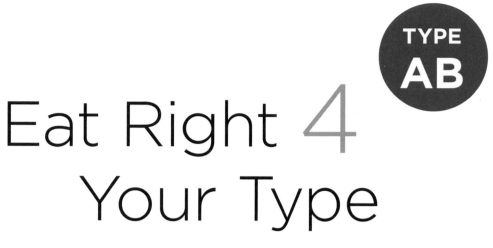

Eat Right 4 Your Type

TYPE
AB

Your Type

PERSONALIZED COOKBOOK

Introduction

Let food be thy medicine,

and medicine be thy food.

—HIPPOCRATES

FOOD HAS THE potential to heal and strengthen our physical bodies, support our recovery from injury and illness, and potentially change our genetic destinies.

Not only does food provide sustenance and nourishment, it provides an opportunity for creative expression and community, whether through developing new recipes or ways to prepare a certain food or in sharing a meal with others. When I wrote *Eat Right 4 Your Type* in 1996, I explored the connections between blood type and diet, and outlined specific nutritional programs for each blood type. Since its publication more than fifteen years ago, I have continued to research and write about the role that foods play in our lives, and I have tried to create support materials and guidance for people who follow the Blood Type Diet®.

In 1998, I wrote *Cook Right 4 Your Type*, which acted as a handbook for my readers, providing recipes, cooking tips, and planning guidelines to help navigate the process of food planning and preparation. I always wanted to take this further as I felt there was an aesthetic quality about food and food preparation that should be reflected in a book, not just with great recipes but also with beautiful, four-color photography that celebrates food. About three years ago, I met Kristin O'Connor. Although she came to see me as a patient, our conversation turned to following the Blood Type Diet, cooking, food preparation, and the work she was doing as a personal chef, food stylist, and food blogger.

I was impressed by her dedication to nutrition and healthy eating, and with her ability to simplify the food-preparation process, which for some people can be quite daunting. Over the ensuing months, as we worked together as doctor and patient, our conversations returned again and again to food. I felt that I had found in Kristin the perfect person to collaborate on a book project that would blend the scientific concepts of the Blood Type Diet with the artistry of cooking to create visually stunning cookbooks specifically designed for each blood type. Kristin has a passion for the Blood Type Diet that is unparalleled, and an encyclopedic knowledge of the food lists for each of the blood types. She is creative and resourceful, and she appreciates and respects the need for food to both taste delicious and be nourishing.

For the past year, I have been enjoying the recipes included in the books, and I have to say that I've been knocked out by how delicious they are. They are also easy to prepare, as I know most of us have limited hours in the day for food planning and preparation. The recipes contained in these books are suitable for individuals or families, as well as for special events and entertaining. Additionally, there are helpful food preparation tips, suggestions for how to organize your kitchen, food storage guidelines, and suggested resources that can make meal planning and preparation easier. My goal has always been to provide accessible information that is easy to incorporate into daily life, and I believe that Kristin has accomplished this.

These cookbooks represent new food and healthy lifestyle possibilities for my readers; they combine the science behind the Blood Type Diet with Kristin's expertise as a chef and believer and follower of these concepts, and package them in a beautiful, four-color format. The recipes contained within are appropriate for your blood type and compliant with the food lists, and they are delicious and made with love—love of food, love of health, and love of sharing this with others on both Kristin's and my part.

I invite you to join us on the continued journey of personalized living. I am confident that you will find a trusted companion in these cookbooks, and one who will make your life richer and healthier as you experiment with the recipes that were developed specifically to be right for your type.

Type AB at a Glance

TYPE AB IS the rarest and newest blood type, found in only 5 percent of the population. The AB blood type evolved out of Types A and B coming together. As a result, those with type AB are fortunate enough to have the strengths of both blood types, but also bear some weaknesses from each parent blood type as well.

AB's dietary profile stems from low stomach acidity, inherited from Type A, which results in slower digestion. Therefore, Type AB, a limited meat eater, benefits from eating multiple, small meals throughout the day, and from separating meats and carbohydrates. This strategy will aid in digestion, help balance insulin, and promote weight loss. Some foods that are highly *Beneficial* for Type AB are lamb, a variety of seafood, soy products, whole grains, and many fruits and vegetables. Those with type AB can enjoy a very balanced diet; however, keep in mind that the approach to maintaining balance is slightly different in this case because small meals and eating proteins away from carbohydrates are ideal. If you are not accustomed to eating proteins in one meal and complex carbohydrates in another, I recommend continuing to make your meal as you normally do and then storing either the protein or the carbohydrate in the refrigerator before you sit down to eat. After a couple of hours, pop the remainder of your meal out of the fridge and heat it up if you like. That way, you don't feel like you are spending your day cooking every couple of hours.

The Blood Type Diet has taken personalized nutrition to a higher level with the introduction of the influence Secretor Status has on our health. Approximately 80 percent of the population are Secretors, which means that the majority of us secrete our blood type antigens in our bodily fluids such as saliva and mucus. As I wrote in *Live Right 4 Your Type*:

> Subtyping your blood, especially your Secretor Status, provides an even greater specificity of identification. Your blood type doesn't just sit inert in your body. It is expressed in countless ways . . . A simple analogy would be a faucet. Depending on the

water pressure, the faucet might pour or dribble . . . In the same way, your Secretor Status relates to how much and where your blood type antigen is expressed in your body.

Being a Secretor means that we can immediately attack viruses, bacteria, and other foreign bodies as they come in contact with our bodies, through secretions in our saliva. Non-Secretors do not have this first line of defense; however, their internal defenses are more powerful than Secretors. All of this means that there are some foods that are suitable for Secretors that may not be for Non-Secretors NS and vice versa. To address this, all recipes in this book are appropriate for Secretors, and additionally we've tagged recipes that are appropriate for Non-Secretors and when possible, substitutions are provided to make the other recipes acceptable and healthful for Non-Secretors.

Those with type AB have a tendency to produce an excess of stress hormones, but often internalize heightened emotions. The AB approach to physical exercise is essential to overall health. Maintaining a balance between intense physical exercise to release stress, and engaging in calming, meditative exercises to center your body and mind will be the key to reducing stress and staying fit. Aim to have an intense workout every other day of the week where you push yourself and work up a sweat followed by a day of meditation, stretching, or calming yoga.

In this book, you will find recipes, menus, and tools specifically designed for the Type AB diet. If you have a SWAMI© Personalized Nutrition Software Program (SWAMI© is a proprietary software program designed to produce a unique, one of a kind diet protocol based on your blood type, a series of biometric measurements, and your personal history. For more information, see page 248 in the Appendix); feel free to modify and substitute accordingly. The goal is to make life easier for you on your Blood Type Diet.

First Things First

Beneficial Foods

Here is a list of basics to keep in your kitchen with the thought that there will be times when meals have to be spontaneous and pretty much thrown together; if you have essentials from your *Beneficial* and *Neutral* lists on hand, no matter what you make, it will be something that is good for you.

Let's Start with the Fridge

Salad Base

Pick your favorite greens or mix it up each time you go to the grocery store to have a great start to a last-minute salad or add crunch to a sandwich, keeping these salad base options in mind:

BENEFICIALS

Dandelion greens   Kale

NEUTRALS

Arugula	Endive	Romaine
Cabbage	Escarole	Spinach
Chicory	Red-leaf lettuce	

Roasted Vegetables

The best thing you could do for yourself is to keep hearty, fresh veggies on hand to roast for dinner, make in bulk to add to a last-minute salad, or to throw in a frittata for breakfast. Roasted vegetables are a terrific leftover to keep on hand. Most vegetables work well when tossed with olive oil and sea salt and roasted in a 375-degree oven for 12 to 20 minutes (depending on the size and density of the vegetables). Here are a few that are both *Beneficial* to Type AB and take well to roasting:

 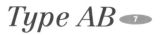

BENEFICIALS

Beets	Eggplant	Sweet potato
Broccoli	Kale	
Cauliflower	Parsnip	

NEUTRALS

Asparagus	Fennel	Squash
Brussels sprouts	Pumpkin	Zucchini
Carrots	Rutabaga	
Celeriac	Turnip	

Keeping a few of these veggies in your fridge each week will come in handy, and is a perfect way to add more *Beneficials* to your diet.

Fruit

Fruit is a perfect snack paired with nuts or nut butters, but you can also use fruit to make desserts or add dried fruit to cereal or salads. Some fruits even work well in savory dishes. Below is a list of *Beneficial* fruit for Type AB:

BENEFICIALS

Cherries	Grapes	Watermelon
Cranberries	Pineapple	
Figs	Plums	

Milk

Keep milk in the refrigerator for smoothies, cereal, some soups, and baked goods. Below are the acceptable milk options for you as a Type AB. Recipes in this book use a combination of the milks listed below but are mostly interchangeable, so if you only have one type of milk on hand, don't hesitate to substitute that for any milk suggested in a recipe.

BENEFICIALS

Goat's milk

NEUTRALS

Almond milk
Nonfat or 2 percent cow's milk

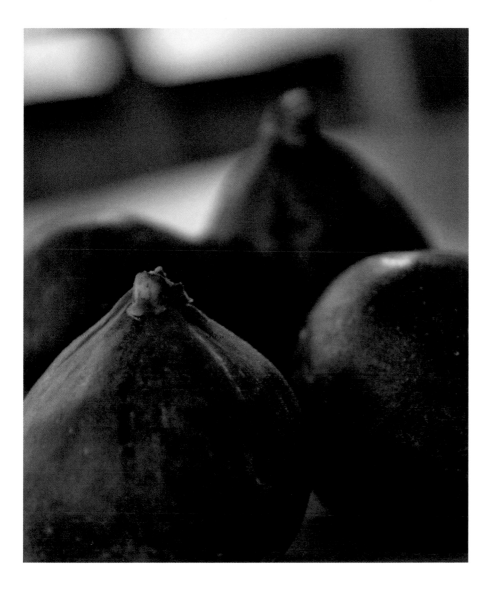

Extras

What about those things we all have hanging around in the door of our fridge, like salad dressings, condiments, and relishes? Toss away those chemical-heavy bottles and jars, and replace them with fresh, tasty, homemade options. Here are a few things that will save your taste buds from boredom:

Carrot-Ginger Dressing NS*
Citrus Dressing NS*
Fresh herbs (basil, oregano, parsley, thyme)

Ghee
Ground flaxseed
Herb Dressing NS*
Honey-Mustard Dressing*

*Recipes provided in books.

Protein

The Type AB diet is based on a combination of animal proteins, vegetable proteins, hearty grains, and fresh, pure fruits and vegetables. Try to diversify your sources of protein. A few *Neutrals* appear on this list, but focus on the *Beneficials* as often as possible.

Please note, it is recommended that all poultry be organic, and all beef be grass-fed and organic.

BENEFICIALS

Beans (lentils, navy beans, pinto beans, red beans)
Eggs
Cheeses (cottage cheese, farmer cheese, feta, kefir, mozzarella, ricotta cheese)
Meat (lamb, mutton, rabbit)
Nut butters (peanut butter). If your SWAMI personalized nutrition report indicates one type of nut that is *Beneficial* above the rest, use that one and make your own butter in the food processor.
Nuts (chestnuts, peanuts, walnuts)
Poultry (turkey)
Seafood (cod, grouper, mackerel, mahimahi, salmon, red snapper, snail, tuna)
Soy (soybeans, tempeh, tofu)

NEUTRALS

Nut butters (almond butter). Almond butter is inexpensive and easily found in supermarkets or natural food stores.

Filling up Your Freezer
Smoothies

Making smoothies is a great alternative for breakfast, or a perfect protein-filled snack. Use fresh fruit in season, and mix in some frozen fruits and vegetables for a thicker consistency. Here are a few *Beneficial* options:

BENEFICIALS

Cherries	Kale
Figs	Pineapple

NEUTRALS

Blackberries	Peaches
Blueberries	Spinach
Dates	Strawberries
Papaya	

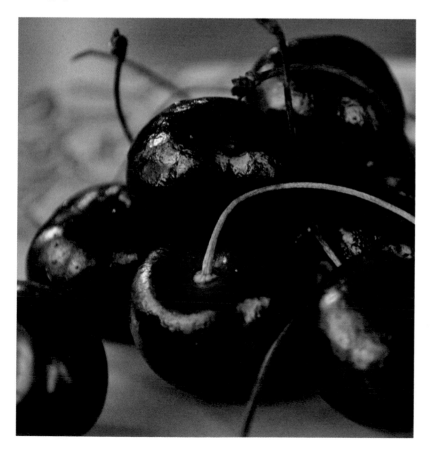

FIRST THINGS FIRST

Type AB 11

Leftovers

It's always helpful to double the recipe when making foods that freeze easily such as:

Chili   Pasta sauce
Cookies   Pesto
Crackers   Sauces
Lasagna   Stew
Muffins

Pesto can be stored in BPA-free ice cube trays for individual servings. On the following pages, you will find more information on safe food storage as well as suggestions for cooking in bulk.

Protein

It is helpful for weeknight dinners to keep at least a few protein options in the freezer. To defrost poultry or seafood, remove from freezer the day before using and place in the refrigerator.

Meat (lamb, rabbit)
Seafood (cod, grouper, mackerel, mahimahi, salmon, red snapper, snail, tuna)
Turkey tenderloins/ground turkey

Time to Get in That Pantry

Snacks

The first thing we all go into the pantry for is to grab a quick bite on the run or to pack a snack to ship off to school with the kids. It is important that these treats are balanced and wholesome, especially to keep your blood sugar balanced. The best way to make that happen is to stock that pantry right. Here are a few staples for Type AB:

Brown rice cakes
Dark chocolate (70 percent or higher)
Dried fruit (apricots, cherries, cranberries, figs, pineapple, prunes, raisins)

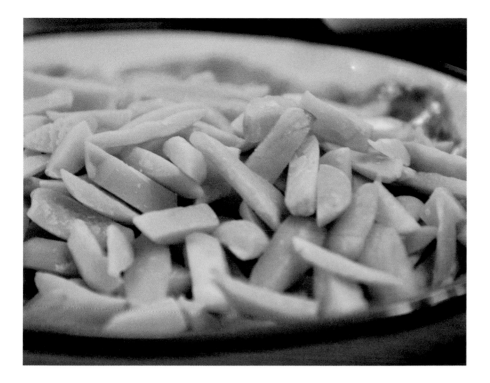

Fresh fruit (cherries, grapefruit, grapes, kiwi, pineapple, plums, watermelon)
Nuts (almonds, peanuts, pecans, macadamia nuts, walnuts)
Peanut butter
Spelt crackers

If you want to prep ahead for those times when you are in a rush, make individual servings of combinations of nuts, dried fruit, and maybe even a little dark chocolate. Store in small, glass, sealable containers and take them in the car, on the plane, or anywhere you are headed.

Bread

As a Type AB, you are among the few who can tolerate wheat. That being said, it is a *Neutral*, and not helpful for weight loss, so you want to focus on grains that are *Beneficial* to your diet. Opt for Ezekiel breads (made from sprouted wheat) or breads made of brown rice, spelt, soy flour, millet, or amaranth. Please note that the commercial version of Ezekiel bread now adds wheat gluten, so be sure to check ingredient lists for potential *Avoid* foods added.

Drinks

Yet another reason you are lucky to be Type AB: red wine is highly *Beneficial* for Non-Secretors and neutral for Secretors. Of course, it's not advisable to drink wine all day, so aside from water, when you want to add a little flavor to your beverage repertoire, dabble in these *Beneficial* teas or fruit juices, plain or with a touch of lemon/lime or mint. In fact, as a Type AB, it is a good idea to start the day with warm water with a squeeze of lemon. There are a few fun recipes for beverages in the recipe section.

BENEFICIALS
Fruit juices (cherry, cranberry, grapefruit, grape, pineapple)
Red wine
Teas (chamomile, echinacea, ginger, ginseng, green, licorice root, rose hip)

NEUTRALS
White wine
Beer

Grains/Legumes

Whole grains and legumes are *Beneficial* to your diet, so try to incorporate them whenever you can. Always keep these ingredients on hand so they are readily available for your use.

BENEFICIALS
Beans (lentils, navy, pinto, red, soybeans)
Whole grains (millet, oat flour, oatmeal, rice, rye flour)

NEUTRALS
Whole grains (barley, couscous, quinoa, wheat)

Seasonings

Making healthy food taste good is non-negotiable. One quick trick is to know the way around your spice cabinet. Herbs and spices are calorie-free and flavor packed. The spices listed below also happen to be terrific for Type ABs. Keep a jar of homemade bread crumbs on hand, too. Additionally, as much as you might like to repress your sweet tooth, it is an unrealistic

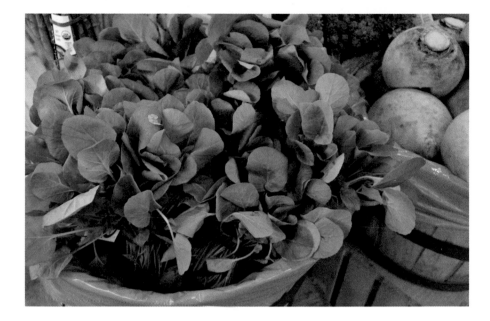

expectation for most, so stock up on natural sweeteners like agave and maple syrup—but use sparingly.

BENEFICIALS

Agave nectar
Basic Bread Crumbs
Blackstrap molasses
Honey
Jam (from allowable fruits)
Jelly (from allowable fruits)
Maple syrup
Mayonnaise
Miso
Olive oil
Soy sauce
Spices (curry, garlic, horseradish, miso, parsley)
Vanilla

NEUTRALS

(basil, bay leaf, caraway, cardamom, carob, chili powder, chive, cinnamon, clove, coriander, cumin, dill, licorice, mustard, nutmeg, paprika, peppermint, rosemary, saffron, sage, sea salt, tamari, tamarind, tarragon, thyme, turmeric)

 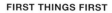

Recipe Ideas for Last-Minute Cooking

Time-Saving Tricks

Make these recipes in bulk and store in your freezer to grab on the go: flax chips, smoothies in individual portions, baked goods, chili, granola, soups, casseroles, sauces, pesto in ice-cube trays, and stews.

When preparing dressings or condiments, double or triple the recipe and store it in the refrigerator for future use. If you are making the recipe with one lemon, you might as well do it with three and save yourself the prep and cleanup again and again.

Utilize Roasted Vegetables

Let's reemphasize here how amazingly useful leftover roasted vegetables can be. Not only are they ready to be thrown into just about any savory dish, but they add tremendous flavor with no effort whatsoever. Here are a few examples where you can toss in roasted veggies and have a tasty new dish:

Casseroles	Quiches
Cold pasta salad	Rice salads
Crêpes	Salads
Frittata	Soufflés
Lettuce wraps	Spring rolls
Omelets	Tacos
Pizza	Vegetable tarts

Review Your Stock

Now that you have the basics, it's time to take a look at some of the *Avoids*. You have lived your whole life eating whatever you want. Now you open your cabinets and think, how do I start over? But the answer is simple: you don't have to. You just have to emphasize the healthy choices that you are now privy to. You should ditch anything that is categorized *Avoids* for your type; listed below are a few places where *Avoids* may be lurking and ready to sabotage your otherwise perfect new diet.

- Fridge: Take inventory of all condiments, sauces, stocks, and other processed foods.

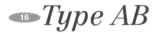

- Pantry: Familiarize yourself with ingredients in your snacks, cereals, pastas, spices, and other foods.
- Freezer: Remove frozen dinners. Just do it. You can be sure they are not doing you any good. Other than that, the same applies here as above—evaluate what you have, and review ingredients just to get yourself acquainted with what you are dealing with.

Once you have done that, take out all questionable foods and line them up on the counter or table. Refer to your Type AB diet in *Eat Right 4 Your Type*, the *Type AB Food*, *Beverage*, *and Supplement Lists*, or, if you have one, refer to your SWAMI personalized nutrition reference book. Check out your *Avoids*, as this will be the most efficient way of eliminating those foods.

Here is a rundown of some of the main offenders:

Corn

Corn has arguably become the source of the greatest debate of the century. The movie *Food Inc.* came out and exposed many people to an understanding about how the mass production of corn has become a national if not global issue. With the introduction of genetically modified organisms (GMOs) or foods that are genetically altered to optimize their growing potential, corn quite literally became another species. As an *Avoid* for Type AB, eliminating corn gives us yet another opportunity to clean our diet. It is used in a wide range of processed goods in this country, making it difficult to avoid altogether. We will do our best to outline where corn is generally hidden, but know, too, that with this diet, it is okay to run into an *Avoid* once in a while without sabotaging your progress. Most ingredients you can't pronounce are corn-based. If you are not acutely sick and are simply using the Blood Type Diet for general health, you only have to be 80 percent compliant to see 100 percent results. How forgiving is that?

The following are a few places corn exists:

Alcohol (some)	Canned vegetables
Artificial flavorings	Caramel color
Artificial sweeteners	Cereal
Ascorbic acid	Cheese spreads
Aspartame	Citric acid
Baked goods	Confectioners' sugar
Baking powder (some)	Corn flour
Canned fruits	Corn starch

 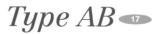

Corn syrup
Fast food
Grits
Hominy
Hydrolyzed vegetable protein
Ice cream (some)
Instant coffee/teas
Ketchup
Licorice
Maize
Malt/malt syrup
Modified food starch
Molasses (some)
Polenta
Popcorn food starch

Prepared mustard (some)
Salad dressings
Salt (iodized)
Soda
Splenda
Sucrose
Sugar (if not cane or beet)
Sweet beverages (containing
    corn syrup)
Taco shells
Tomato sauce (with corn syrup)
Vitamins (some)
Xanthan gum
Yeast (some)
Yogurt (with corn syrup)

Meat

Although there are some red meats that are on your *Beneficial* list, beef is not one of them. This will either be something you are excited or disappointed about. If you are currently a big beef eater, don't worry about it for now. Unless you have a very acute illness that requires immediate, strict adherence to the diet, it is okay to ease into it. Take your time and instead of trying to eliminate foods, focus on the foods that ARE *Beneficial* to you and try to eat them as often as possible.

Wheat

Although Type AB does not have to be gluten-free, it is most *Beneficial* for you to be as wheat-free as possible, both for optimal weight loss and health. Luckily for you, there are plenty of non-wheat options to cook with and buy as healthier substitutions. Spelt or brown rice breads are readily available in health food stores and online, and they are very close to the texture and taste of wheat breads. Wheat exists in a surprising number of places, many where you would never suspect:

Baking powder (some)
Beer
Blue cheese (some)
Brewer's yeast

Bread crumbs
Breaded fish
Breads
Broth (some)

Bulgur
Candies (some)
Caramel color (some)
Cereal
Chewing gum
Cookies
Cold cuts (some)
Corn bread
Couscous
Crackers
Croutons
Dumplings
Farina
Flavored extracts (some)
Food starch or modified food starch (some)
Graham flour
Gravy
Hot dogs
Hush puppies
Hydrolyzed plant protein
Hydrolyzed vegetable protein
Ice cream (some)
Kamut
Malt (flavoring, and vinegar)
Matzo
Meatballs
Meat loaf
"Natural flavor" (either soy or gluten)
Pancakes
Pasta
Pastries
Pie crust
Pitas
Pizza crust
Potato chips (some)
Pretzels
Salad dressings
Seitan
Semolina
Soups
Soy sauce
Spice mixtures (some)
Syrup
Tamari
Teriyaki sauce
Textured vegetable protein
Wheat protein
Wheatgrass
Worcestershire sauce

Chicken

Chicken seems to be the most difficult exclusion for Type ABs. The challenging part of no longer eating chicken is figuring out options when eating out. In your own kitchen, chicken can easily be replaced with turkey in most recipes. Because Type ABs are made to have balanced diets, however, you can see that there are many options still available when dining out at a restaurant.

Vinegar

You are a Type AB and thus not vinegar friendly. You might be cringing at the thought of living sans-vinegar. But don't fret: We will give you recipes to fill the void. For now, let's get it out of your kitchen—out of sight, out of mind. So, the big question is, where does vinegar lurk when the word *vinegar* is not in the name—as in balsamic, red wine, apple cider, or rice wine vinegars?

Chili sauces	Prepared mustard
Cocktail sauce	Relishes
Ketchup	Salad dressings
Mayonnaise	Steak sauce
Olives	Soy sauce
Pickled vegetables	Worcestershire sauce
Pickles	Steak sauce
Prepared horseradish	

Peppers (Spice)

Although most vegetables are healing for your body, peppers are not among them. There are many varieties of peppers, from sweet bell peppers to spicy chipotle so this is just a little reminder to be wary of anything spicy. The only two exceptions to this rule are paprika (a spice made from red bell peppers) and pimientos (a mild red pepper).

The Rest

Other than what is listed above, it will be straightforward to determine what to take out of your cabinets/fridge/freezer. Take the time to go through your list of *Avoids* and remove them from your house. If you have canned goods and nonperishables, you can donate to your local food bank. To find a food bank in your area, go to: http://feedingamerica.org.

Now you are ready to go to the store and grab a few essentials to fill in the gaps.

How to Read These Recipes

This cookbook is designed to be as practical and helpful to the Blood Type Dieter as possible. We took into consideration that many families could be cooking for multiple blood types or preparing meals for friends with varying blood types. In order to make doing so practical, each of the *Eat Right 4 Your Type Cookbooks* contains the same or similar recipe ideas with different executions to suit the needs of each blood type. You will find the recipe titles almost identical in each book; however, ingredients and methods might vary quite a bit. There are many recipes that are *Beneficial* across the board and are marked with an (A/B/AB/O) to identify that they are universal to every type. For example, every blood type has a pancake recipe; however, the Type A recipe has *Beneficial* grains that might be on the *Avoid* list for other blood types, so each recipe contains different flours. Every recipe is also written to contain as many *Beneficial* foods as possible, while understanding that taste is still of the utmost importance. After all, you are not going to be inclined to dive into a kale cookie, but you won't be able to resist Pasta Carbonara with Crispy Kale. The point is, we want you coming back for more each time to see that eating right for your blood type is as far from sacrifice as is indulging in a bar of chocolate.

As you make your way through this book, you will notice that once in a while there is a highlighted section called "Featured Ingredient." There are several ingredients used in this book that you may not have come across before, some that are *Beneficial* for your diet and some that are *Beneficial* for your taste buds. In an effort to familiarize you with these ingredients, there is a brief summary explaining a little about what that ingredient is, and how or why it is used. Don't be afraid to experiment with unfamiliar territory.

Many people who follow the Blood Type Diet have come to my office or used the tests on my website (www.dadamo.com) to create a specific diet plan. If you have done that, you have a SWAMI personalized nutrition plan that may vary slightly from the general Type AB diet because it takes into consideration family and medical history, Secretor Status, and GenoType. (The GenoType is a further refinement of my work in personalized nutrition. It uses a variety of simple measurements, combined with blood type data, to classify individuals as one of six basic Epigenotypes: The Hunter, Gatherer, Teacher, Explorer, Warrior, and Nomad types.) Due to the variations in *Beneficial, Neutral,* and *Avoid* foods, there may be some recipes containing ingredients that do not suit you as an individual. Please do not skip these recipes entirely. There is always a way to make quick and easy substitutions. As a quick piece of advice, however, vegetables can be easily swapped out— leafy greens for other leafy greens, specific type of beans for another, or in some cases, simply omitted from the recipe if it is not a star component.

You will see that recipes are also tagged according to Secretor Status. Some recipes are not appropriate for Non-Secretors but are fine for Secretors (see legend on the following page). In most instances when this is the case, there are simple substitutions to adapt the recipe for Non-Secretors. In a few cases, however, there will be no easy substitution and the recipe will be an *Avoid* altogether for a Type AB Non-Secretor.

In many of the recipes in this book, you will see sea salt written as "sea salt, to taste," and might be wondering what that means or how much to add. Salt can make or break your dish. But, if you add too much, there is no going back. Try adding a little at a time, taste, and add more if needed. What is *a little*? Well, start with pinching a bit between your fingers and sprinkling it into your dish, give it a minute to incorporate, and then taste. If you were to measure a pinch, it would be a little less than ⅛ of a teaspoon.

As you know at this point, one of the major changes for people following the Type AB diet is becoming chicken-free. Throughout the book, recipes that could use chicken as a star ingredient are replaced with tofu, tempeh, or some kind of turkey. If you have the reaction to the idea of tofu or tempeh that most people do the first time they see it, this may be a very unappealing swap for you. Please give these ingredients a try. The best part about tofu is that it is a blank canvas for any of your favorite flavor combinations. When marinated in soy, honey, and ginger, for example, and then seared in a bit of olive oil, tofu is transformed into a delicious and desirable meal, one you will certainly not shun the next time around.

Remember to read each recipe in its entirety beforehand to ensure you know how much time it will take and if there are any ingredients you will need to buy ahead of time. Finally, enjoy making, eating, and sharing these recipes.

RECIPE LEGEND:

- An * is used when a recipe ingredient needs further instruction, substitutions, or comment. This information is found at the bottom of a recipe.
- All recipes are appropriate for Type AB Secretors.
- (NS) represents a recipe that is appropriate for Type AB Secretors as well as Non-Secretors.
- Recipe ingredients that are NOT appropriate for Type AB Non-Secretors (NS) are notated with appropriate acceptable substitutions within recipe ingredients.

A REVIEW OF THE FOOD LISTS

Throughout this book we refer to a number of places to find the comprehensive food lists for the Blood Type Diet. Here's a recap of where you can find the lists so you can use the one that is right for you:

- *Eat Right 4 Your Type*, which provides the entry point into the Blood Type Diet.

- *Live Right 4 Your Type*, which incorporates the value of the Secretor Status.
- *Blood Type AB Food, Beverage, and Supplement Lists from Eat Right 4 Your Type*, a handy pocket guide with the basic food lists.
- *Change Your Genetic Destiny* (originally published as *The Geno-Type Diet*, which provides a further refinement of the diet by using blood type, secretor status, and a series of biometric measurements to further individualize your food lists).
- SWAMI Personalized Nutrition Software is designed to harness the power of computers and artificial intelligence, using their tremendous precision and speed to help tailor unique, one-of-a-kind diets. From its extensive knowledge base, SWAMI can evaluate over 700 foods for over 200 individual attributes (such as cholesterol level, gluten content, presence of antioxidants, etc.) to determine if that food is either a superfood or toxin for you. It provides a specific, unique diet in an easy-to-read, user friendly format, complete with food lists, recipes, and meal planning.

Breakfast

Breakfast recipes were written with diversity in mind so that you do not end up eating the same thing every day. The idea here is to alternate: one day eggs, the next quinoa or granola, and so on, in order to keep providing your body with different nutrients each day. You will probably notice the biggest changes in these recipes are the types of flour used. Don't be intimidated; try one simple recipe like Spelt Pancakes to get your feet wet, and then move on to the rest. Once you have the new flour on hand, the rest is just like any other recipe.

Quinoa Muesli (NS)

½ cup quinoa

½ cup water

½ cup (2 percent) cow's or goat's milk

¼ teaspoon sea salt

2 tablespoons dried cherries

1 tablespoon dried cranberries

2 tablespoons slivered almonds

2 tablespoons chopped walnuts

¼ teaspoon cinnamon

2 teaspoons maple syrup

¼ cup crunchy rice cereal

1. Rinse quinoa. Combine in a small saucepan with water, milk, sea salt, cherries, and cranberries, and bring to a boil. Reduce heat and simmer 10 minutes, turn off the heat, and let sit an additional 4 to 5 minutes. Quinoa will absorb all the water and become light and fluffy when done.

2. In the meantime, toast almonds and walnuts in a dry skillet for about 2 minutes or until slightly golden brown. Watch nuts carefully; because of their high fat content, they have a tendency to burn easily.

3. Fluff cooked quinoa with a fork and add toasted nuts, cinnamon, and maple syrup. Top with crunchy rice cereal and add more milk, if desired.

4. Serve immediately.

▶ SERVES 2

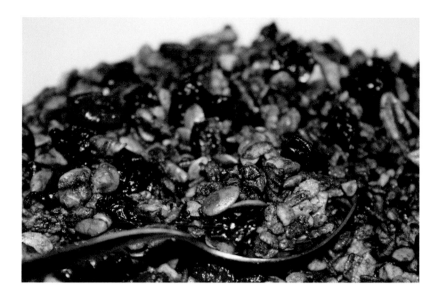

4 cups crispy rice cereal

1 cup chopped walnuts

1 cup chopped pecans

¼ cup whole flaxseed

¼ cup blackstrap molasses

2 teaspoons olive oil

1 tablespoon agave

⅛ teaspoon sea salt

¼ cup water

1 cup halved dried cherries

½ cup halved dried cranberries

1. Preheat oven to 350 degrees. Line a baking sheet with parchment paper and set aside.

2. In a large bowl, combine rice cereal, walnuts, pecans, and flaxseed. Set aside.

3. Combine molasses, olive oil, agave, salt, and water in a small saucepan. Heat mixture over medium heat for 2 minutes, whisking until smooth.

4. Pour the liquid over granola mixture, toss to coat, and spread onto prepared sheet pan. Bake 10 minutes.

5. Reduce oven temperature to 300 degrees. Stir granola, and place back in the oven. Bake an additional 25 minutes.

6. Toss granola with cherries and cranberries.

7. Serve warm, or cool fully and store in an airtight, glass container for up to 2 weeks or in the freezer for up to 2 months.

▶ MAKES 24 (¼-CUP) SERVINGS

Granola–Nut Butter Fruit Slices NS

3 tablespoons peanut butter

⅓ cup granola*

¼ teaspoon cinnamon

Sea salt, to taste

1 pear

1 apple

1 lemon

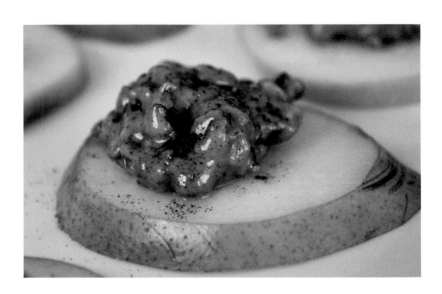

1. Stir peanut butter, granola, and cinnamon (if using), until granola is evenly coated, and season with sea salt to taste, set aside.

2. Thinly slice fruit into ¼-inch rounds. Cut lemon in half and rub cut side on fruit pieces to prevent browning. Spoon 1 to 2 teaspoons of the granola mixture on fruit and enjoy.

*See Blackstrap-Cherry Granola NS recipe (page 27).

▶ SERVES 4

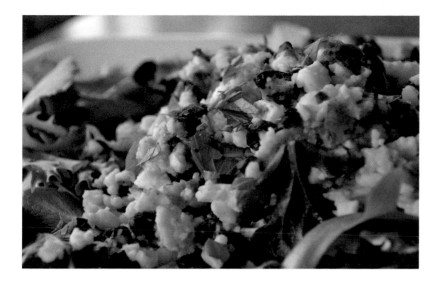

dressing:

½ teaspoon mustard powder

1 tablespoon olive oil

1 tablespoon lemon juice

1 tablespoon onion, grated

Sea salt, to taste

salad:

2 teaspoons olive oil

½ cup cooked or canned pinto beans, drained and rinsed

3 large hard-boiled eggs

¼ cup grated mozzarella cheese

1 tablespoon chopped parsley

2 cups mixed baby greens

Sea salt, to taste

1. Whisk together dressing ingredients in a small bowl until combined, and set aside.

2. Heat olive oil in a small skillet over medium heat. Toast pinto beans for 2 to 3 minutes until warm and slightly crunchy.

3. Remove eggs from shells, and use a fork to break apart in a bowl. Add beans, cheese, and parsley to eggs and toss with dressing. Season with sea salt to taste and serve over mixed baby greens.

▶ SERVES 4

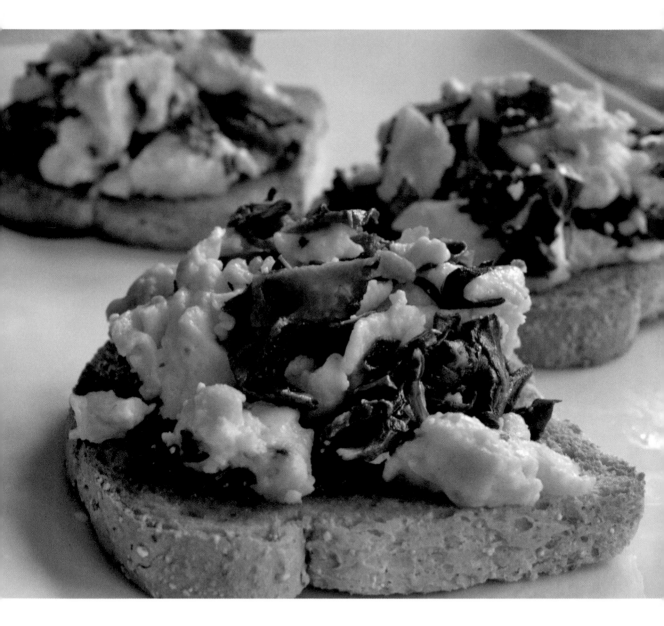

Turkey Bacon–Spinach Squares 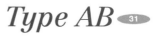 NS

3 strips nitrate- / preservative-free turkey bacon

3 eggs

3 egg whites

2 teaspoons olive oil

2 cups fresh spinach

Sea salt, to taste

¼ cup Cheddar cheese

4 slices Ezekiel or spelt bread, toasted

1. Heat a large skillet over medium and coat with nonstick cooking spray.

2. Once the skillet is hot, add bacon and cook 3 to 4 minutes, flip, and cook an additional 2 to 3 minutes for crispy bacon. Remove from pan, crumble, and set aside.

3. Whisk eggs and egg whites in a small bowl. In the same skillet used for the bacon, add olive oil and reduce heat slightly. Add spinach, sauté 2 minutes, and season with sea salt. Pour eggs over spinach, cooking gently until done, about 2 minutes. Remove from heat and add reserved bacon and cheese.

4. Spoon mixture on toast and serve immediately.

▶ SERVES 4

tip: If the bacon is not as crispy as you'd like, drizzle a touch of olive oil into the pan.

featured ingredient

turkey bacon (nitrate- /preservative-free)

Not all turkey bacon is the same. There are many types/brands on the market, but most are artificially derived and loaded with salt, preservatives, and full of nitrates . . . all things you absolutely do not want to be eating. There are a few companies that make turkey bacon without these unhealthy and artificial additives; they can be found at your local natural food store and in some mainstream grocery stores.

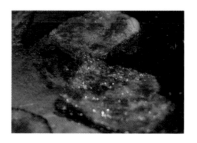

Type AB 31

Swiss Chard and Eggplant Frittata

2 teaspoons ghee

¼ cup finely diced Spanish onion

1 cup diced eggplant

3 cups chopped Swiss chard

3 large eggs

3 large egg whites

2 tablespoons spelt or oat flour

½ teaspoon sea salt

1 teaspoon fresh basil

1 teaspoon olive oil

¼ cup toasted pine nuts

1. Preheat oven to 375 degrees.

2. Melt ghee in a heatproof sauté pan over medium heat. Sauté onion, eggplant, and Swiss chard for 4 to 5 minutes.

3. While vegetables cook, whisk together eggs, egg whites, flour, salt, and basil in a large bowl. Add olive oil to the skillet and pour egg mixture over vegetables. Cook for 1 minute.

4. Transfer sauté pan to oven and bake 6 to 8 minutes, or until firm and edges are golden brown. Top with pine nuts and serve warm.

▶ SERVES 4

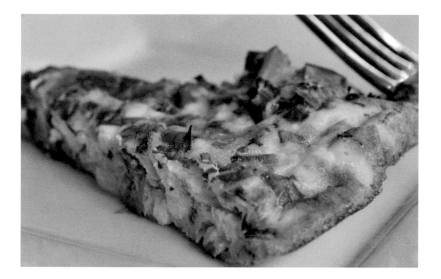

Broccoli-Feta Frittata

1 head broccoli

½ teaspoon sea salt, divided

1 tablespoon plus 2 teaspoons olive oil

3 large eggs

2 large egg whites

⅓ cup crumbled feta

½ cup chopped spinach

¼ cup finely diced chives

2 teaspoons spelt flour

1 tablespoon chopped oregano

1. Preheat oven to 375 degrees.

2. Dice broccoli into bite-size pieces and place in a single layer on a baking sheet. Sprinkle with sea salt and 1 tablespoon olive oil. Bake 15 minutes, remove from oven, and set aside. Turn oven to Broil setting.

3. In a medium-size bowl, whisk eggs, egg whites, feta, spinach, chives, flour, oregano, and salt until well combined.

4. Heat remaining 2 teaspoons olive oil in a heatproof medium skillet over medium heat. Add egg mixture and broccoli to pan. Cook 1 to 2 minutes, lifting the side of the eggs gently with your spatula to encourage uncooked egg to run down into the bottom of the skillet. (If the handle of your skillet is rubber, wrap tightly with tinfoil to prevent melting.)

5. Place skillet under broiler for 2 minutes, or until the eggs set and brown very slightly on the edges.

6. Serve warm.

▶ SERVES 4

Maple-Sausage Scramble

2 cups asparagus spears

2 teaspoons olive oil, divided

¼ cup finely chopped white onion

3 cups chopped kale

⅓ cup diced vine-ripened tomatoes

½ pound ground turkey sausage

1 tablespoon maple syrup (NS omit maple syrup)

3 large eggs

2 large egg whites

1 tablespoon water

Sea salt, to taste

¼ cup diced kefir cheese

1. Cut asparagus spears in thirds. Heat 1 teaspoon olive oil in a medium skillet over medium heat. Sauté onion, kale, asparagus, and tomatoes for 8 to 10 minutes, until vegetables are tender and cooked through. Remove from skillet and set aside.

2. In same skillet, heat remaining 1 teaspoon olive oil. Brown turkey sausage, breaking into bite-size pieces, until cooked through, about 5 to 6 minutes. Drizzle with maple syrup and stir to combine. Add sausage to vegetables and set aside.

3. Whisk eggs and egg whites with water and salt to taste and add to skillet, reducing the heat to medium-low. Stir gently with a heat safe spatula until firm and cooked through. Return sausage mixture back to skillet, and toss to combine.

4. Top with kefir cheese and serve warm.

▶ SERVES 4

1. In a large sauté pan, heat olive oil over medium heat and add onions and fennel. Sauté 3 to 4 minutes, or until tender. Remove from heat and let cool to room temperature, about 10 minutes.

2. While vegetables cool, place ground turkey in a large bowl and add fennel seed, paprika, salt, garlic, pear, maple syrup, and cooled vegetables. Use your hands to incorporate all ingredients, but do not over mix.

3. Form meat into small, hot dog–shaped links. Cook 8 to 10 minutes over medium heat in a skillet sprayed with nonstick olive oil spray until meat is browned on all sides, and the inside of the sausage is no longer pink.

4. Serve warm alone or alongside scrambled eggs for a protein-packed breakfast.

▶ SERVES 4

Homemade Turkey Breakfast Sausage (NS)

2 teaspoons olive oil

½ cup finely diced onion

½ cup finely diced fennel

1 pound ground turkey

1 teaspoon fennel seed

1 teaspoon paprika

1 teaspoon sea salt

1 clove garlic, minced

½ cup finely diced Bosc pear

2 teaspoons maple syrup (NS omit maple syrup)

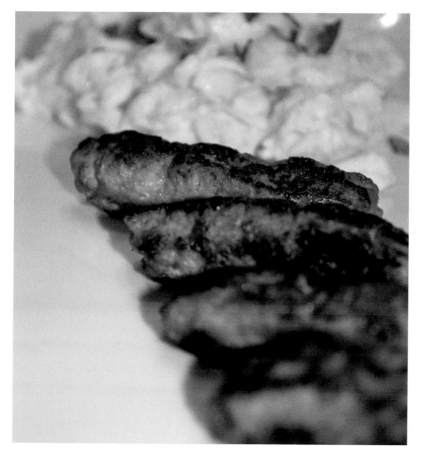

Savory Herb and Cheese Bread Pudding NS

2 teaspoons olive oil

1 teaspoon ghee

2 cups diced onion

2 cups quartered cremini mushrooms

2 cups diced zucchini

6 cups torn kale

Sea salt, to taste

8 cups (sprouted wheat or spelt) bread cubes, about 10 slices

1 cup (2 percent) cow's or goat's milk

1 cup Vegetable Stock*

4 large eggs, beaten

1 teaspoon finely chopped fresh rosemary

1 teaspoon finely chopped fresh sage

1 teaspoon fresh thyme

1 cup mozzarella cheese

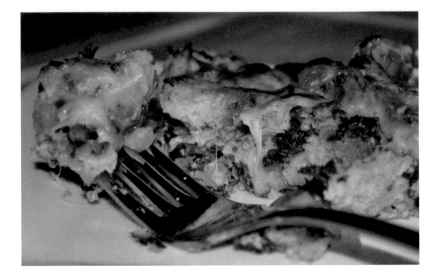

1. Preheat oven to 350 degrees. Grease bottom and sides of a 9" × 11" baking dish with nonstick cooking spray and set aside.

2. Heat olive oil and ghee in a large skillet over medium heat. Sauté onion, mushrooms, zucchini, and kale just until tender, about 5 to 6 minutes. Season with salt, to taste, and set aside.

3. Spread bread cubes on a baking sheet in a single layer. Toast for 3 to 4 minutes until slightly golden brown. Toss in a large bowl with vegetables.

4. Whisk together milk, stock, eggs, rosemary, sage, and thyme. Pour over bread and vegetables and toss. Transfer mixture to prepared baking dish. Top with mozzarella cheese and bake, covered, for 35 minutes. Uncover, and bake an additional 10 minutes.

5. Serve warm.

*See Vegetable Stock NS recipe (page 221).

▶ SERVES 12

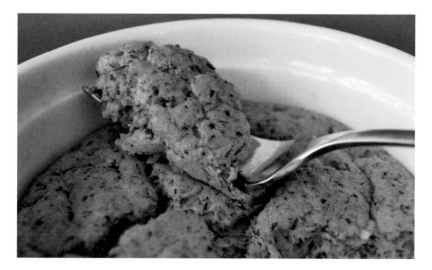

Kale and Zucchini Soufflé NS

1. Preheat oven to 350 degrees. Spray 4 (12-oz.) ramekins with nonstick cooking spray and set aside.

2. In a medium saucepan melt ghee over medium heat, and whisk in flour. Gradually add milk and stock, whisking continuously until thickened, about 3 to 4 minutes. Once mixture is thick and resembles the consistency of yogurt, remove from the heat and cool completely.

3. Grate kale and zucchini in a food processor, and strain excess liquid through cheesecloth or paper towel. Place vegetables in a bowl and whisk in egg yolks, basil, cheese, and cloves. Fold milk mixture into pureed vegetables, and set aside.

4. In a dry, glass bowl, beat egg whites with a hand mixer until they form stiff peaks. Fold egg whites, one-third at a time, into the vegetables. Divide mixture evenly among prepared ramekins. Set ramekins on a baking dish and place on the middle rack in your oven, fill the baking dish halfway with hot water. Bake for 45 minutes or until tester comes out clean.

5. Serve immediately.

*See Vegetable Stock NS recipe (page 221).

▶ SERVES 4

1 tablespoon ghee

2 tablespoons brown rice or spelt flour

½ cup (2 percent) cow's or goat's milk

½ cup Vegetable Stock*

2 cups packed chopped kale

2 cups chopped zucchini

2 large egg yolks

¼ cup basil

¼ cup grated Gruyère cheese

⅛ teaspoon ground cloves

4 large egg whites, room temperature

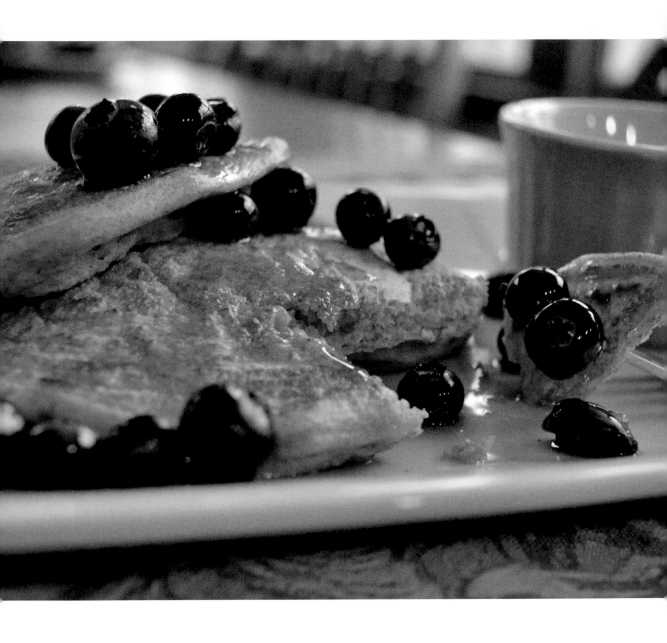

1. Combine flours, baking powder, and salt in a large bowl, and set aside.

2. In a separate bowl, whisk eggs, milk, and olive oil. Add to flour mixture and stir until well combined and free of lumps.

3. Heat a large skillet over medium heat and spray with nonstick cooking spray. Spoon ¼ cup batter into and cook 1 to 2 minutes per side. Repeat with remaining batter.

4. Serve warm.

5. If making a large batch, keep warm in the oven at 200 degrees, draped with a slightly damp paper towel.

▶ **SERVES 4**

¾ cup spelt flour

¼ cup oat flour

2 teaspoons baking powder

½ teaspoon sea salt

2 large eggs

1 cup (2 percent) cow's or goat's milk

2 tablespoons olive oil

featured ingredient

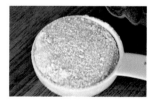

spelt flour

Spelt is an ancient grain related to wheat with a slightly nuttier flavor and a greater amount of nutrients. It can be used as a direct substitution in almost any recipe calling for wheat flour. Although spelt contains gluten, it does not seem to be a problem for people who cannot tolerate wheat. Spelt can be purchased in a variety of forms, from the whole grain to flour, pasta, and bread. Store spelt in the refrigerator to retain the maximum benefits of its nutritional value.

Cinnamon-Oat Crêpes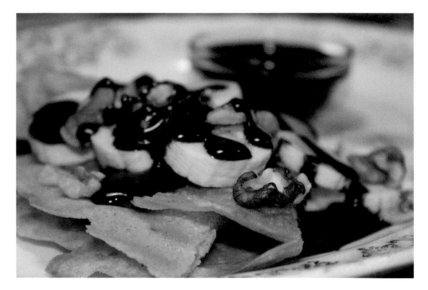

NS

⅔ cup oat flour

⅓ cup spelt flour

¼ teaspoon sea salt

¼ teaspoon cinnamon

1¼ cups (2 percent) cow's or goat's milk

2 large eggs

1 tablespoon plus 1 teaspoon melted ghee, divided

1. In a medium bowl, whisk together flours, sea salt, and cinnamon.

2. In a separate bowl, whisk milk, eggs, and 1 tablespoon ghee; add to flour mixture and whisk until well blended. Cover and let sit in the refrigerator for 1 hour.

3. Heat a large sauté pan over medium. When the pan is hot, brush remaining 1 teaspoon ghee evenly across the bottom of the pan. Using a ¼-cup measure, scoop batter into pan and quickly turn in circular motions to spread the batter into a very thin layer. Let cook 1 minute or until the batter firms and edges lift slightly off the pan. Use an offset spatula to flip and cook 1 additional minute. Repeat with remaining batter. Keep cooked crêpes warm by wrapping in a damp kitchen towel in a 200-degree oven.

4. For an indulgent treat top with sliced bananas, walnuts, and Chocolate Syrup*.

*See Chocolate Syrup NS recipe (page 218).

▶ SERVES 4

featured ingredient

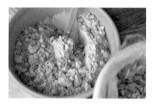

oat flour

Oats have a delicious, creamy flavor, and add smooth texture to baked goods. You can make oat flour yourself by grinding quick-cooking oats in your food processor until fine. Naturally rich in fiber, one benefit of including oats in your diet is their ability to satiate your appetite, so you will not feel hungry soon after your meal. Because oats do not contain gluten, if used in baked goods without a self-rising flour like wheat or spelt, they will not work quite as well. This is why most of the recipes in this book call for a combination of oat and spelt flours.

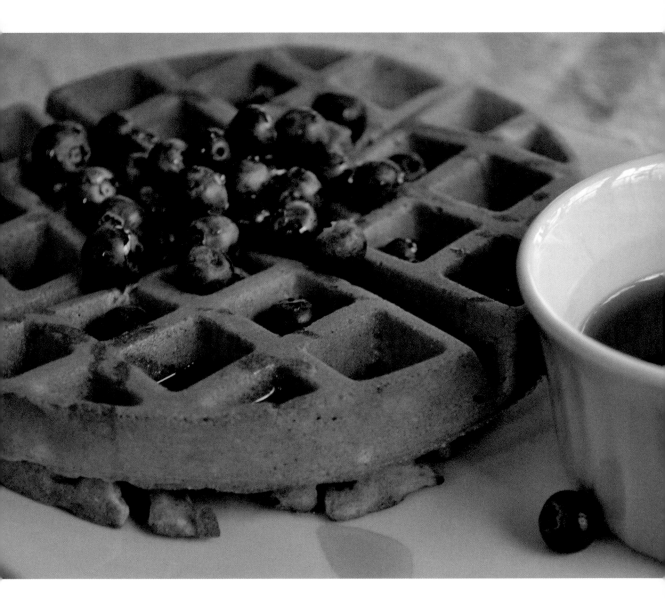

Wild-Rice Waffles (NS)

1. Preheat waffle maker according to manufacturer instructions.

2. In a large bowl, whisk together flours, flaxseed, salt, baking powder, and cinnamon until well combined.

3. In a separate bowl, combine eggs, milk, olive oil, and applesauce. Add to dry ingredients, and mix until free of lumps. Fold in cooked rice.

4. Spoon batter into waffle maker just to the rim, close, and cook according to settings on your waffle maker. Waffles should be firm with a slightly crunchy exterior and soft interior.

5. Serve warm.

▶ SERVES 4

1½ cups spelt flour

½ cup oat flour

2 tablespoons flaxseed

½ teaspoon sea salt

2 teaspoons baking powder

¼ teaspoon cinnamon

2 large eggs

2 cups (2 percent) cow's or goat's milk

2 tablespoons olive oil

2 tablespoons applesauce

1 cup cooked wild rice

featured ingredient

flaxseed

Flaxseeds are small with a hard, smooth surface and are packed with omega-3 fatty acids as well as manganese, fiber, and other nutrients. Foods rich in omega-3s are a healthy addition to any diet, and provide anti-inflammatory benefits for Type ABs specifically in their ability to fight cancer and diabetes. Flaxseed can be added to smoothies, baked goods, or even used as a topping on salads. When submerged in warm water, flaxseed binds together with the water and forms a gelatin that is helpful in gluten-free baking, and if drunk will help keep you "regular."

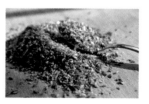

Pumpkin Muffins with Carob Drizzle (NS)

2 cups spelt flour

1 cup oat flour

2 teaspoons baking powder

½ teaspoon baking soda

½ teaspoon sea salt

1 teaspoon ground cinnamon

⅛ teaspoon ground cloves

½ teaspoon ground ginger

1 (15-oz.) can organic pumpkin puree

½ cup honey

2 large eggs

½ cup (2 percent) cow's or goat's milk

topping:

¼ cup rolled oats

⅓ cup finely chopped pecans

½ teaspoon ground cinnamon

1 tablespoon honey

1 tablespoon almond or light olive oil

¼ cup Carob Extract™*

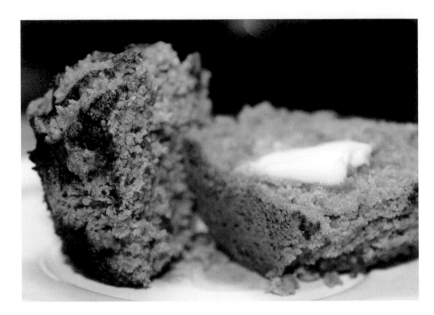

1. Preheat oven to 350 degrees. Line a 12-cup muffin tin with paper liners, and set aside.

2. In a large bowl, stir together spelt, oat flour, baking powder, baking soda, salt, cinnamon, cloves, and ginger until well combined.

3. In a separate bowl, whisk pumpkin, honey, eggs, and milk until well combined. Add pumpkin mixture to the flour mixture and stir to incorporate. Divide batter evenly among prepared muffin tins.

4. Place oats, pecans, cinnamon, honey, and oil in a small bowl, and toss with a fork to combine. Divide topping evenly among muffins, and drizzle with Carob Extract™.

5. Bake 20 to 25 minutes or until a toothpick inserted into muffin comes out clean.

▶ SERVES 12

*Information about purchasing Carob Extract™ can be found in Appendix II: Products (page 247).

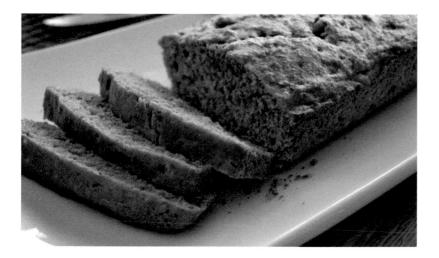

Pear-Rosemary Bread NS

½ cup diced fresh pear

¾ cup spelt flour

½ cup oatmeal flour

1 tablespoon finely chopped fresh rosemary

½ teaspoon fine-grain sea salt

2 teaspoons baking powder

2 large eggs

¼ cup agave

¼ cup extra virgin olive oil

⅓ cup chopped walnuts

1. Preheat oven to 350 degrees. Grease a 8½" × 4½" loaf pan with olive oil spray and set aside.

2. Set pears out on a paper towel to drain excess water.

3. Whisk flours, rosemary, salt, and baking powder in a large bowl to combine.

4. In a separate bowl, whisk eggs, agave, and olive oil until well combined. Add the wet ingredients to the flour mixture and stir to combine. Fold in chopped walnuts and drained pears.

5. Spoon batter into prepared loaf pan. Bake 30 to 35 minutes or until cake tester inserted into middle of loaf comes out clean.

▶ SERVES 10

tip: Refillable spray cans are widely available, so fill with allowable oil and use as nonstick spray.

Cherry Scones (NS)

½ cup dried cherries, halved

1 cup spelt flour, plus more for rolling

½ cup oat flour

¼ cup almond flour

2 teaspoons baking powder

½ teaspoon sea salt

4 tablespoons cold ghee

¼ cup (2 percent) cow's or goat's milk

1 large egg

1 teaspoon lemon zest

⅓ cup agave

topping:

2 tablespoons agave

2 tablespoons almond flour

1. Preheat oven to 350 degrees. Line a baking sheet with parchment paper and set aside.

2. Place dried cherries in a small bowl and cover with hot water for 10 minutes to rehydrate. Remove, pat dry, and set aside.

3. In a large mixing bowl, combine flours with baking powder and salt.

4. Cut ghee into small cubes, and cut into the flour mixture using a pastry cutter or two butter knives until mixture resembles coarse corn meal. Add cherries, mixing just until they are evenly distributed throughout the flour.

5. In a separate bowl, whisk milk, egg, lemon zest, and agave until well combined. Fold the milk mixture into the dry until well combined. Dough will be thick and slightly sticky. Use extra flour to form the dough into a ball. Gently place on a floured surface and using your hands, pat dough into a rectangular shape about 1 inch thick. Using a sharp knife, cut the dough horizontally once and then into thirds vertically, to makes 6 squares. Cut each square again at an angle to make 12 triangles. Gently place each scone on prepared baking sheet. Brush the tops evenly with agave and almond flour.

6. Bake 20 to 22 minutes until firm and bottoms are lightly browned. Serve warm or cool completely and store in a cool, dry place overnight.

7. Scones can be frozen for up to 1 month. Reheat at 200 degrees for 10 minutes.

▶ SERVES 12

EAT RIGHT FOR YOUR TYPE PERSONALIZED COOKBOOK

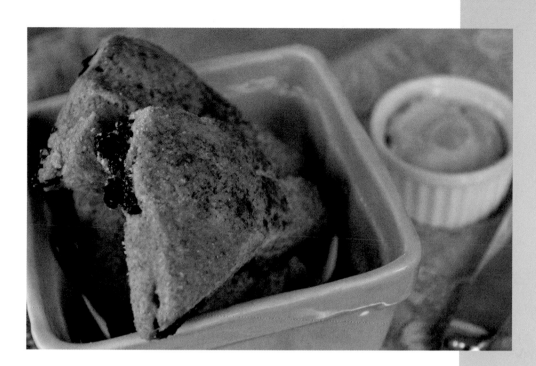

tip: Keeping all ingredients—and your mixing bowls—cold creates a flaky texture in your scones.

featured ingredient

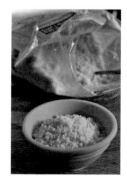

almond flour

To make almond flour, blanched almonds are ground into a fine meal. Almond flour is great to use in baked goods such as cookies, muffins, or dense cakes. It lends a sweet flavor, and adds protein and healthy fats. Almond flour adds a soft, grainy texture that helps to make cookies crispier and gives cake additional texture.

Blueberry-Walnut Muffins

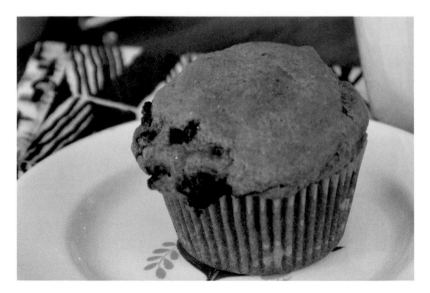

1½ cups spelt flour

1 cup oat flour

½ teaspoon salt

2 teaspoons baking powder

1 teaspoon baking soda

½ teaspoon cinnamon

2 large eggs

½ cup agave

½ teaspoon lemon zest

3 tablespoons light olive oil

½ cup applesauce

½ cup plus 2 tablespoons nonfat cow's or goat's milk

½ cup chopped walnuts

1 cup (fresh or frozen) organic blueberries

1. Preheat oven to 350 degrees. Line a 12-cup muffin tin with paper liners and set aside.

2. In a large bowl, combine flours, salt, baking powder, baking soda, and cinnamon. Set aside.

3. In a separate bowl, whisk eggs with agave, lemon zest, olive oil, applesauce, and milk.

4. Add the wet ingredients to the dry ingredients, stirring to combine. Fold in walnuts and blueberries. Spoon batter evenly into prepared muffin tins and bake for 25 to 28 minutes, or until a cake tester or toothpick inserted into muffin comes out clean.

▶ SERVES 12

Lunch

Each lunch recipe is written to provide a balance between vegetables and varying types of proteins while staying light on complex carbohydrates. Recipes that are more dominantly vegetable or protein include suggestions for a tasty complement of the other.

Navy Bean Hummus and Feta Sandwich (NS)

2 slices brown rice or Ezekiel bread

½ teaspoon olive oil

Large-grain sea salt, to taste

2 tablespoons Navy Bean Hummus*

1 (1¼-inch-thick) slice feta cheese

¼ cup arugula

1. Toast bread lightly, just until honey brown and drizzle one side of each slice with olive oil and a scant sprinkling of sea salt.

2. Smear hummus on the olive oil side of one piece of toast, then top with feta and arugula. Place the second piece of toast oil side down and slice in half.

3. Serve immediately.

*See Navy Bean Hummus NS recipe (page 165).

▶ SERVES 2

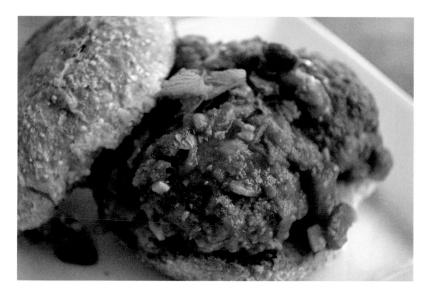

Lamb Meatball Subs

1. Preheat oven to 400 degrees. Line a baking sheet with parchment paper and set aside.

2. Place lamb in a large bowl and add onion, mint, sea salt, curry, egg, and bread crumbs. Gently combine all ingredients with clean hands. Try not to overwork the meat because it will get too tough.

3. Roll meatballs into golf ball–size pieces and place on prepared baking sheet about 2 inches apart. Bake for 20 minutes or until golden brown and cooked through.

4. While meatballs cook, prepare tomato sauce. Heat olive oil in a high-sided skillet over medium heat,. Once hot, sauté onion and garlic for 5 to 6 minutes. Add tomatoes and bring to a boil, reduce to a gentle simmer, and cook 10 to 15 minutes. Add salt to taste.

5. When meatballs are done cooking, add to sauce and toss to coat.

6. Spoon meatballs onto buns and serve warm.

*See Basic Bread Crumbs recipe (page 222).

▶ SERVES 4

1 pound lean ground lamb

¼ cup onion, grated

⅓ cup finely chopped fresh mint leaves

¼ teaspoon sea salt

1 teaspoon curry powder

1 large egg

5 tablespoons bread crumbs*

sauce:

2 teaspoons olive oil

1 cup diced white onion

2 cloves garlic, minced

5 vine-ripened tomatoes, chopped

Sea salt, to taste

4 brown rice/millet or spelt buns

Fish Fillet Sandwich

1 pound cod

¼ teaspoon sea salt

1 large egg, slightly beaten

½ cup spelt flour

1 teaspoon garlic powder

1 tablespoon olive oil

4 brown rice or spelt buns

1 cup shredded romaine lettuce

sauce:

1 (5.5-oz.) container thick Greek yogurt

1 tablespoon minced onion

Sea salt, to taste

1 tablespoon chopped fresh dill

2 teaspoons lemon zest

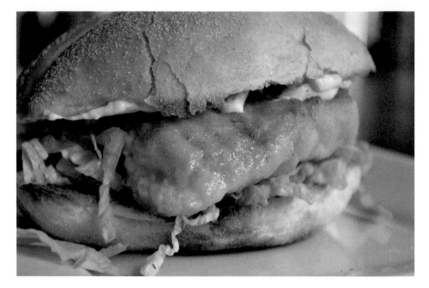

1. Season cod with sea salt and slice into 4 individual fillets. In a large, flat-bottomed bowl, add beaten egg. Combine flour and garlic powder in a second bowl. Dip each cod fillet into the egg mixture and then into flour mixture. Dust off excess flour and place onto a clean plate.

2. In a large, high-sided skillet, heat olive oil over medium heat. Once hot, add fish fillets, keeping 2 inches of space between each one. Cook about 4 minutes per side or until center is flaky and opaque.

3. Toast buns, and set aside.

4. Combine all sauce ingredients in a medium bowl. Spoon yogurt sauce on each half of the bun, and top with romaine and cooked fish.

▶ SERVES 4

tip: Keep an eye on the fish while it cooks to ensure it does not burn. You may need to flip the fish twice to make sure this does not happen. If more oil is needed, add 1 teaspoon at a time.

EAT RIGHT FOR YOUR TYPE PERSONALIZED COOKBOOK

1. Preheat oven or toaster oven to 200 degrees.

2. Heat olive oil in a medium skillet over medium heat. Cook bacon for 1 to 2 minutes per side, until crispy. Drain on paper towel and keep warm in oven; this will help the bacon crisp up further.

3. In same skillet, heat remaining oil and sauté spinach over medium heat for 1 to 2 minutes, just until leaves are wilted.

4. Spread ghee evenly on one side of each piece of bread. Place bacon, spinach, and cheese on unbuttered side of bread and top with a second piece of buttered bread. Toast in a skillet over medium heat until lightly browned on each side and cheese has melted.

5. Slice in half and serve warm.

▶ SERVES 2

2 teaspoons olive oil, divided

4 strips (nitrate- and preservative-free) turkey bacon

4 cups spinach

4 teaspoons ghee

4 slices Ezekiel bread

½ cup shredded mozzarella cheese

Greens and Beans Salad

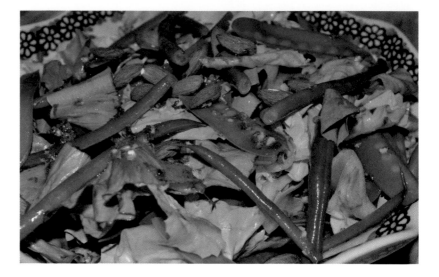

1 head escarole

½ cup cooked or canned pinto beans, drained and rinsed

2 cups snap peas

4 cups string beans

dressing:

1 tablespoon chopped mint

1 tablespoon fresh lime juice

⅛ teaspoon cumin

1 clove garlic, minced

½ teaspoon honey (NS substitute agave)

¼ cup olive oil

Sea salt, to taste

1. Wash escarole and pat dry. Tear into bite-size pieces, and place in a large serving bowl. Top with pinto beans and set aside.

2. Bring a large pot of water to boil. Cook snap peas and string beans for 3 minutes, drain, and shock in a large bowl of ice water to stop the cooking process. Lay the peas and beans on a kitchen towel to dry, and add to escarole.

3. Place all dressing ingredients in a small bowl and whisk to combine. Drizzle over salad and serve.

▶ SERVES 4

EAT RIGHT FOR YOUR TYPE PERSONALIZED COOKBOOK

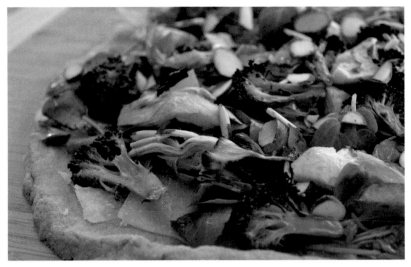

Salad Pizza NS

Store-bought, precooked spelt crust with allowable grains

¼ cup shaved hard goat cheese

1 head broccoli

1 teaspoon olive oil

Sea salt, to taste

dressing:

1 tablespoon fresh lemon juice

1 teaspoon onion, minced

1 tablespoon olive oil

2 teaspoons chopped fresh oregano

2 cups watercress

1 cup sliced cucumber

1 tablespoon blanched, slivered almonds

1. Preheat oven to 375 degrees.

2. Top pizza crust with cheese. Bake for 3 minutes, just until the cheese melts slightly. Remove from oven and set aside. Increase oven temperature to 400 degrees.

3. Cut broccoli in to bite-size florets and place on a baking sheet, and toss with olive oil and sea salt. Bake for 20 minutes. Remove and let cool.

4. While the broccoli cooks, whisk together dressing ingredients until combined.

5. Toss dressing with watercress, cucumber, broccoli, and almonds. Top crust with salad mixture and serve cold.

▶ SERVES 4

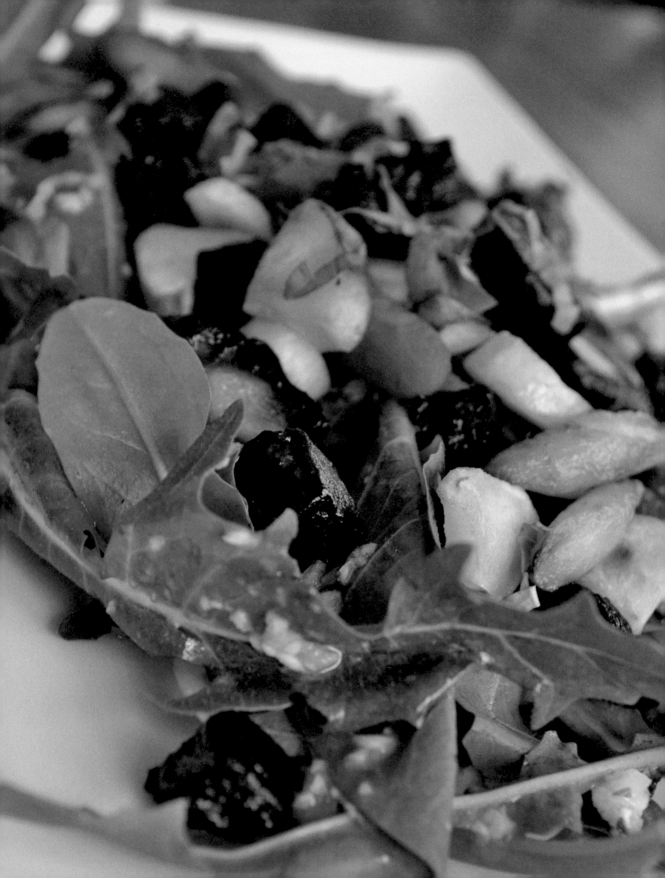

1. Preheat oven to 375 degrees.

2. Peel beet, carrots, and parsnips. Dice vegetables into ½-inch cubes. Toss with olive oil and season with sea salt. Spread in a single layer on a baking sheet and bake for 55 to 60 minutes, tossing halfway through.

3. To prepare dressing, add horseradish to a bowl with olive oil, basil, lemon juice, and sea salt, to taste, and whisk all ingredients to combine.

4. Toss dandelion greens in a large bowl with horseradish dressing, top with roasted vegetables, and serve.

▶ SERVES 4

tip: If you cannot find tri-colored carrots, plain carrots will work just fine.

1 raw beet

3 small, tri-colored carrots

2 medium parsnips

2 teaspoons olive oil

2 bunches dandelion greens

Sea salt, to taste

dressing:

¼ cup fresh finely grated horseradish

¼ cup olive oil

1 tablespoon fresh basil

2 tablespoons fresh lemon juice

Sea salt, to taste

Roasted Tomato Greek Salad NS

1 pint heirloom cherry tomatoes

1 teaspoon olive oil

Sea salt, to taste

6 cups torn romaine lettuce

½ cup Spanish green olives

½ cup crumbled feta cheese

dressing:

1 tablespoon fresh oregano

2 tablespoons fresh squeezed lemon juice

3 tablespoons olive oil

Sea salt, to taste

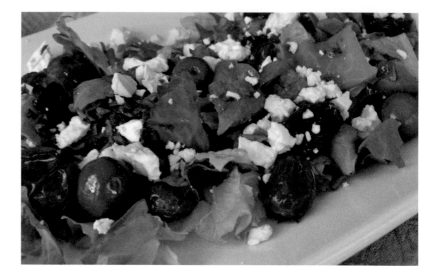

1. Preheat oven to 375 degrees.

2. Place tomatoes on a baking sheet. Drizzle with olive oil, sprinkle with sea salt, and bake for 35 minutes on the top rack of oven. Tomatoes will collapse and slightly char when fully cooked. Remove from oven and let cool.

3. In the bottom of a large bowl, whisk dressing ingredients together and set aside.

4. Place lettuce in a serving bowl. Add roasted tomatoes, olives, feta cheese, and dressing, and toss to combine.

▶ SERVES 4

1. Peel outer leaves of radicchio, and discard the first couple of leaves. Continue peeling inner leaves gently, snapping at the base to maintain the integrity of each leaf. Clean with cold water and let dry on a kitchen towel.

2. Flake salmon into a bowl, and add chives, salt, peas, and apples.

3. Whisk together honey, oregano, lemon juice, lime zest, and olive oil. Drizzle over salmon mixture, and spoon mixture into prepared radicchio cups.

▶ SERVES 2

1 head radicchio

½ pound salmon, cooked

3 tablespoons diced chives

½ teaspoon sea salt

½ cup cooked peas

½ cup finely diced apples

1 teaspoon honey

1 teaspoon chopped fresh oregano

Juice of 1 lemon

Zest of 1 lime

¼ cup olive oil

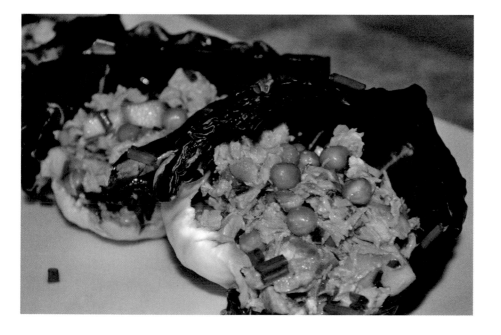

Baked Falafel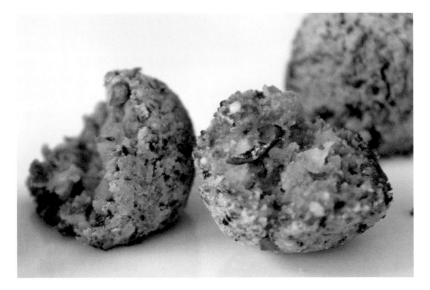

NS

1½ cups raw pinto beans (not canned or precooked)

1 tablespoon olive oil, divided

½ cup chopped parsley

2 tablespoons spelt flour

1 cup chopped onion

2 cloves garlic, minced

¼ teaspoon ground coriander

¼ teaspoon ground cumin

½ teaspoon sea salt

1. Soak dry beans overnight in cold water, drain, and rinse.

2. Boil presoaked beans for 30 minutes, drain, and rinse. Beans should remain slightly firm; this will help falafel's texture. Set beans in a single layer on a paper towel to dry.

3. Preheat oven to 350 degrees. Brush a baking sheet with 1 to 2 teaspoons olive oil, and set aside.

4. In a food processor, combine beans, parsley, flour, onion, garlic, coriander, cumin, and salt. Pulse until ingredients form a thick paste. Using a tablespoon measure, scoop mixture into the palm of your hand, roll into a ball, and place on prepared baking sheet. Repeat with remaining falafel mixture. Brush remaining olive oil on the tops of falafel balls and bake for 25 minutes.

5. Increase oven temperature to 400 degrees and bake an additional 15 minutes. When done, falafels will be firm, slightly moist, and gently browned on the bottoms.

6. Serve on top of Roasted Tomato Greek Salad (page 58).

▶ SERVES 4

Raw Kale Salad with Zesty Lime Dressing NS

1. Wash kale and dry on kitchen towels. Strip kale off the woody stems by holding the stem with one hand and wrapping finger and thumb of the other hand around the stem and quickly pulling down. Discard stems and tear leaves into bite-size pieces. Place in a large bowl and set aside.

2. Heat olive oil in a medium skillet over medium heat. Sauté onion for 3 to 4 minutes. Add raisins, and cook for 5 minutes. Remove from heat and toss with raw kale.

3. Whisk dressing ingredients in a small bowl. Drizzle over kale salad and toss to coat.

▶ SERVES 4

1 bunch kale
2 teaspoons olive oil
1 large white onion, sliced
½ cup raisins

dressing:
2 tablespoons olive oil
Juice of 2 limes
1 clove garlic, minced
⅛ teaspoon ground cumin
Sea salt, to taste

tip: For added protein, serve with leftover or chilled baked salmon, roasted chicken, or beans.

Crunchy Green Bean and Beet Spring Rolls with Sweet Cherry Dip (NS)

2 teaspoons olive oil

2 cups green beans

¼ cup finely chopped onion

1 cup sliced cooked beets

¼ cup julienned fresh basil

2 tablespoons slivered almonds

Sea salt, to taste

4 rice paper wraps

sweet cherry dip:

⅓ cup (no sugar added) cherry jam

1 tablespoon fresh grated ginger

1 tablespoon onion, finely diced

1 teaspoon agave

Juice of ½ lemon

Sea salt, to taste

1. Heat olive oil in a medium skillet over medium heat. Sauté green beans and onion for 3 to 4 minutes. Remove from heat and toss with beets, basil, and almonds, and season with sea salt, to taste. Set aside.

2. Pour hot water halfway up a large, flat-bottomed bowl. One at a time, submerge rice paper wraps in water until they soften and become pliable, about 30 seconds. Rice paper will be delicate, so be gentle. Place rice wrap on a placemat or cutting board and place a small spoonful of the vegetable mixture down the center of the rice paper. Roll the sides of the rice paper over the vegetables first and then pull the top over the vegetables and continue to roll. Slice in half and repeat with remaining filling and rice papers. Set aside.

3. In a small saucepan, combine all sauce ingredients over low heat. Stir for 1 to 2 minutes, until warmed through and smooth.

4. Serve wraps with cherry dip.

▶ SERVES 2

featured ingredient

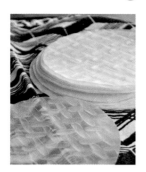

rice paper wraps

Typically found in Asian markets, rice paper is used to make spring rolls and thanks to its increase in popularity, can now be found at most natural or health food stores. It is made of rice and water and when dried resembles stiffened parchment paper that looks pretty inedible! When soaked in warm water, however, rice paper transforms to a pliable, tender state and can be used as a delicate wrap for fresh, delicious flavors that get wrapped inside like a burrito. Rice paper comes in packages of fifty to one hundred papers and cost close to nothing, so it is a great, low-calorie, low-budget addition to your culinary repertoire.

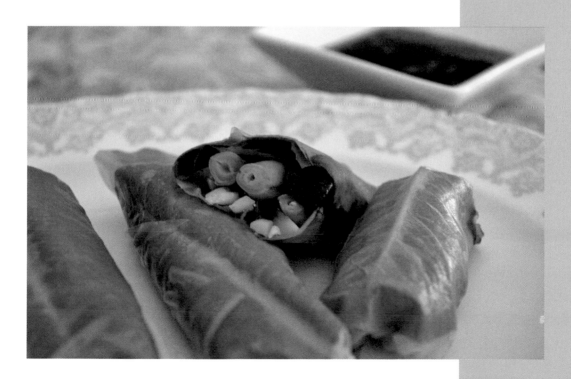

Feta, Spinach, and Broccoli Pie (NS)

crust:

1 cup spelt flour plus more for rolling

¼ teaspoon sea salt

4 tablespoons ghee, chilled

4–5 tablespoons ice water

filling:

2 teaspoons olive oil

4 cups baby spinach

2 cups red kale

1 tomato, diced

1 cup broccoli florets

2 shallots, diced

1 cup feta cheese

2 large eggs

⅓ cup Vegetable Stock*

2 tablespoons fresh thyme

Sea salt, to taste

1. Preheat oven to 375 degrees.

2. Whisk together spelt flour and salt. Cut cold ghee into small pieces and add to flour mixture. Using a crossing motion with two butter knives or a pastry cutter, incorporate ghee into the flour until the mixture resembles coarse cornmeal. Add water, 1 tablespoon at a time, just until the dough comes together but is not sticky. Gather dough in your hands and knead until dough becomes smooth and pliable. Small pieces of ghee should still be visible. Try not to overwork the dough or it can become tough. Cover with plastic wrap and refrigerate 1 hour.

3. Roll dough out on a floured surface until about 12 inches in diameter and approximately ⅛ inch thick. Place dough into a 9-inch pie plate, gently press into the pan, and pinch edges between two fingers to create crimped edges.

4. Par-bake crust for 15 minutes. ("Par-bake" means that you are partially baking the crust before adding the filling.)

5. Prepare filling while crust bakes. Heat olive oil in a large skillet over medium heat. Sauté spinach, kale, tomato, broccoli, and shallots for about 4 minutes, just until vegetables are tender. Remove vegetables from heat, transfer to a large bowl, toss with feta, and let cool.

6. In a separate bowl, whisk eggs, stock, thyme, and salt. Pour over cooled vegetables and mix to combine.

7. Pour filling into par-baked pie crust and bake 30 minutes or until filling is firm.

8. Serve warm or cold (if serving cold, let cool and then place in refrigerator until ready to eat).

*See Vegetable Stock NS recipe (page 221).

▶ SERVES 6

Pinto Bean Stew NS

2 teaspoons olive oil

1 cup diced onion

1 celery root, peeled and diced into ¼-inch cubes

2 cups sweet potato, peeled and diced into ½-inch cubes

2 cans organic pinto beans, drained and rinsed

1½ cups Vegetable Stock*

1 clove garlic

1 sprig sage

4 sprigs thyme

1 teaspoon sea salt

2 cups snow peas

¼ cup feta cheese

1. In a large Dutch oven, heat olive oil over medium heat. Add onions and celery root, and sauté for 4 to 5 minutes. Add sweet potato and sauté an additional 2 to 3 minutes. Add beans, broth, garlic, sage, thyme, and salt and bring to a gentle boil.

2. Reduce heat, cover, and simmer 30 minutes.

3. Add snow peas and cook an additional 5 minutes.

4. Crumble feta cheese over stew and serve warm.

*See Vegetable Stock NS recipe (page 221).

▶ SERVES 4

EAT RIGHT FOR YOUR TYPE PERSONALIZED COOKBOOK

Dinner

The bulk of recipes in this book are in this section. Here you will find a variety of dishes from pasta to seafood to all-in-one-pot meals. Most recipes are simple to make and get on the table in no time, but there are a few meant for lazy Sundays as well.

Roasted Tomato and Broccoli Mac and Cheese NS

1 large head broccoli

4 plum tomatoes

5 sprigs thyme, divided

1 tablespoon olive oil

Sea salt, to taste

¾ cup bread crumbs*

1 tablespoon plus 2 teaspoons ghee, divided

2 tablespoons brown rice or spelt flour

1 cup (2 percent) cow's or goat's milk

2 cups Vegetable Stock*

2 sprigs fresh sage

1 pound brown rice or quinoa elbow pasta

1 cup shredded mozzarella cheese

½ cup cubed fresh mozzarella cheese

1. Preheat oven to 375 degrees.

2. Cut broccoli and tomatoes into bite-size pieces. Place in a single layer on a baking sheet, sprinkle with thyme, and drizzle with olive oil and salt. Bake for 30 minutes, until the vegetables are tender and slightly browned. Remove from oven and set aside.

3. Toss bread crumbs with 2 teaspoons of melted ghee and a pinch of sea salt, and set aside.

4. Melt remaining 1 tablespoon ghee in a saucepan over medium-low heat and whisk in rice flour until well combined into a paste. Let the roux cook for 2 to 3 minutes; this will help take away the raw flour taste. Gradually add milk and stock to flour mixture, whisking after each addition until mixture is smooth and without lumps. Add sage and bring to a boil, whisking constantly. Reduce to a simmer, cooking until the roux thickens, about 10 minutes. Add salt, to taste.

5. Cook pasta according to package instructions (if using brown rice pasta, cook 3 to 4 minutes short of package instructions). Drain pasta and pour into a 14" × 9" casserole dish. Toss with roasted vegetables. Cover pasta with sauce and shredded mozzarella cheese, gently tossing with pasta to incorporate throughout the dish. Top with reserved bread crumbs and fresh mozzarella.

6. Bake 20 to 25 minutes, until mac and cheese is hot and bubbling and bread crumbs are golden brown.

*See Basic Bread Crumbs recipe (page 222). See Vegetable Stock NS recipe (page 221).

▶ SERVES 6

Pasta Carbonara with Crispy Kale (NS)

1. Bring a large pot of salted water to a boil. Cook pasta 4 minutes short of package recommendations. Drain, reserving ½ cup cooking water.

2. While pasta cooks, heat olive oil in a large, high-sided skillet over medium heat. Sauté onion for 4 to 5 minutes, until translucent and tender. Remove from skillet and set aside.

3. In same skillet, sauté turkey bacon until browned, about 2 to 3 minutes. Remove turkey bacon and set aside.

4. In same skillet, add asparagus and kale, sauté until tender, about 3 to 4 minutes. Toss bacon back into the skillet and reduce heat to low.

5. In a bowl, whisk together eggs, egg yolks, milk, ricotta cheese, and salt. Slowly pour hot pasta cooking water into the egg mixture to temper the eggs.

6. Remove skillet from heat and add pasta. Pour over egg mixture while stirring. The heat from the pasta will gently cook the eggs and create a sauce.

7. Gently fold asparagus, kale, onion, and bacon into pasta mixture and serve warm.

▶ SERVES 6

1 pound brown rice or spelt pasta

2 teaspoons olive oil

½ cup diced onion

4 slices nitrate- / preservative-free turkey bacon, diced

2 cups asparagus, sliced on the bias

3 cups sliced red kale

2 large eggs

2 large egg yolks

¼ cup (2 percent) cow's or goat's milk

½ cup ricotta cheese

Sea salt, to taste

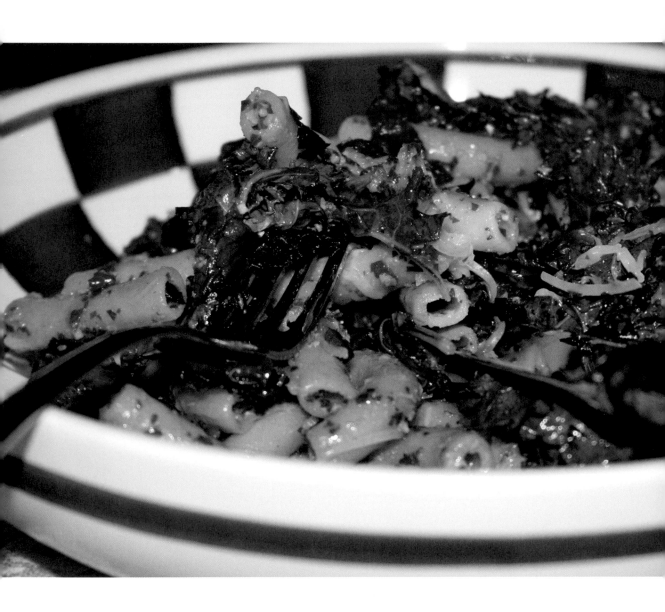

1. Preheat oven to 375 degrees.

2. Snap asparagus spears close to the bottom, and discard the woody stems. Cut into bite-size pieces and toss in a large bowl with 1½ bunches of kale stripped from stems and torn into large, bite-size pieces. Toss with 2 teaspoons olive oil and a pinch of salt.

3. Place vegetables on a baking sheet and bake for 12 minutes, or until vegetables are tender and kale has slightly crispy edges. Remove and set aside. Reduce oven temperature to 200 degrees.

4. Cook pasta according to package instructions (if using brown rice pasta, cook 4 to 5 minutes short of package instructions).

5. Placing remaining half bunch of kale, ½ cup olive oil, lemon juice, walnuts, garlic, and salt in a food processor, and pulse until smooth. Spoon into a bowl and set aside.

6. Heat remaining 1 teaspoon olive oil in a medium skillet over medium heat. Cook bacon until crispy, about 2 minutes per side. Wrap in a paper towel and keep warm in oven until ready to serve; this will make the bacon extra crispy.

7. Drain pasta and place in a large bowl. Immediately toss with pesto, cheese, peas, and roasted vegetables. Crumble bacon, sprinkle on top of pasta, and serve warm.

▶ SERVES 6

1 bunch asparagus

2 large bunches kale, divided

½ cup plus 3 teaspoons olive oil, divided

Sea salt, to taste

1 pound spelt or brown rice pasta

Zest and juice of 1 lemon, divided

½ cup walnuts

2 cloves garlic, minced

3 slices nitrate- / preservative-free turkey bacon

½ cup Gouda cheese, grated

2 cups cooked peas

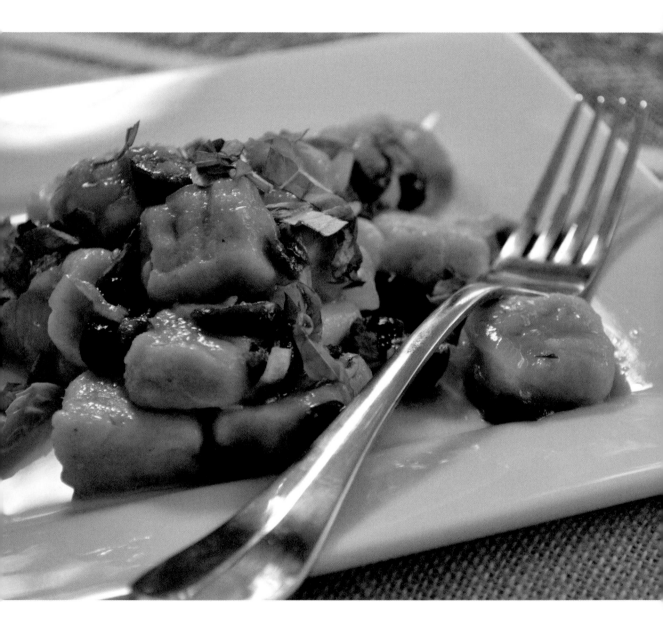

1. Mash boiled sweet potatoes with a fork or potato masher until smooth and creamy.

2. In a large bowl, combine mashed sweet potatoes with remaining gnocchi ingredients. Using your hands, gently form dough into a ball. If the dough is too sticky, sprinkle brown rice flour on top. Working with a handful of dough at a time, roll on a floured surface into long, ¾-inch cylinders. Repeat with remaining dough.

3. Use a sharp knife to slice the cylinders into 1-inch pieces. Roll each piece gently over the back of a fork, to make indentations in the gnocchi.

4. Bring a large pot of salted water to a gentle boil. Drop gnocchi into the water in small batches, being careful not to crowd the pot. The gnocchi will float to the top when they are finished cooking, about 2 to 3 minutes. Remove from pot with a slotted spoon, and transfer to a baking sheet until all gnocchi are cooked.

5. While gnocchi are cooking, heat olive oil and ghee in a saucepan over medium heat. Sauté shallots for 2 to 3 minutes and add stock, lemon juice, and cranberries.

6. Toss gnocchi with sauce just to coat, garnish with basil, and serve warm.

*See Vegetable Stock NS recipe (page 221).

▶ SERVES 4

gnocchi:

2 cups sweet potato, boiled

¾ cup brown rice or spelt flour

¼ cup millet flour

1 teaspoon sea salt

1 large egg, beaten

¼ teaspoon freshly ground nutmeg

sauce:

1 tablespoon olive oil

1 teaspoon ghee

¼ cup finely diced shallots

½ cup Vegetable Stock*

1 tablespoon lemon juice

¼ cup dried cranberries

½ cup torn fresh basil

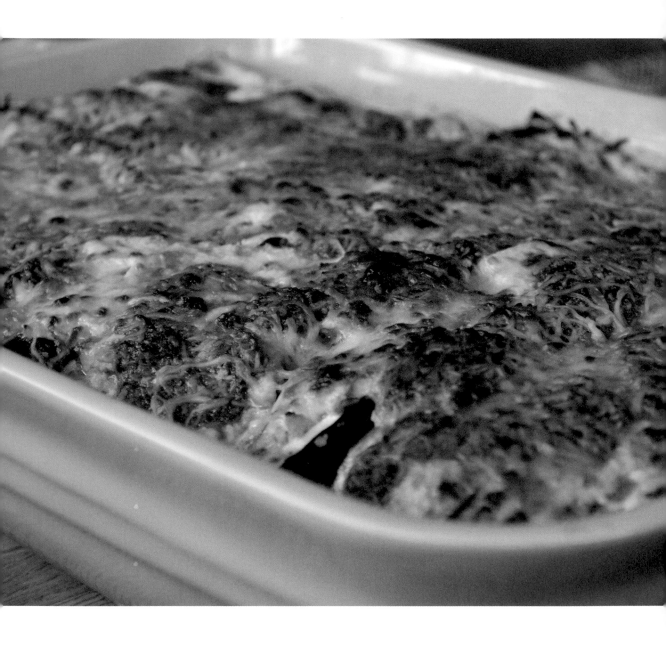

1. Preheat oven to 375 degrees.

2. Trim ends off zucchini and slice in 4 long pieces, about ¼-inch thick.

3. Place zucchini and mushrooms in a single layer on baking sheets. Drizzle evenly with 2 tablespoons olive oil and 1 teaspoon sea salt. Roast on the top rack of oven for 20 minutes.

4. While the vegetables cook, heat remaining 2 teaspoons olive oil in a medium skillet over medium heat. Sauté onion for 8 to 10 minutes, until tender and translucent. Add spinach and sauté 1 minute, just until spinach wilts. Remove from heat.

5. In a large bowl, stir together ricotta cheese, walnuts, egg, cloves, and reserved spinach mixture.

6. Remove vegetables from the oven and let cool while you make the pesto. Reduce oven temperature to 350 degrees.

7. Place all pesto ingredients in a blender and pulse until smooth.

8. Spoon a thin layer of pesto into the bottom of a 9" × 11" baking dish. Top with a layer of roasted zucchini, a layer of ricotta mixture, ½ cup mozzarella cheese, pesto, and mushrooms, followed by ricotta, pesto, remaining zucchini, remaining ricotta, remaining pesto, and remaining mozzarella cheese.

9. Bake for 25 minutes until cheese is melted and slightly browned.

10. Serve warm.

▶ SERVES 6

5 medium zucchinis

6 portabella mushrooms

2 tablespoons plus 2 teaspoons olive oil, divided

1½ teaspoons sea salt, divided

1 cup finely diced onion

4 cups packed baby spinach

2 cups part-skim ricotta cheese

½ cup finely chopped walnuts

1 large egg

Dash cloves

pesto:

2 cups packed baby spinach

2 cups packed basil

½ teaspoon sea salt

2 cloves garlic

¼ cup lemon juice

¼ cup olive oil

¼ cup walnuts

2 tablespoons water

1 cup shredded mozzarella cheese

Grilled Radicchio and Walnut-Spinach Pesto (NS)

infused oil:

Zest of ½ lemon

⅓ cup olive oil

⅛ teaspoon mustard powder

½ teaspoon cumin seeds

2 cloves garlic, smashed

pesto:

¼ cup plus 2 tablespoons toasted almonds, divided

2 tablespoons olive oil

2 tablespoons chopped fresh sage

1 cup chopped spinach

2 tablespoons lemon juice

1 teaspoon lemon zest

½ teaspoon sea salt

1 tablespoon water

¾ pound spinach spelt pasta

2 heads radicchio

½ cup kefir cheese, cut into 1-inch dice

1. In a small skillet, combine all infused oil ingredients. Cook on low heat for 15 minutes. Remove from heat and set aside.

2. In a food processor or mini-chopper, combine ¼ cup almonds, olive oil, sage, spinach, lemon juice, lemon zest, sea salt, and water. Pulse until mixture is pureed and resembles a thick sauce. Set aside.

3. Bring a large pot of salted water to a boil. Cook pasta according to package instructions.

4. While the pasta cooks, heat a grill pan over medium heat and brush with infused oil. Peel outer layers of radicchio and cut into quarters. Brush each piece with infused olive oil and grill 1 minute per side or until radicchio becomes tender and slightly wilted.

5. Drain pasta and toss with pesto and cheese in a large serving bowl. Top with grilled radicchio and remaining 2 tablespoons toasted almonds. Serve immediately.

▶ SERVES 4

tip: Store infused oil in a sealed glass container in a cool, dry place for up to 1 week. The oil is great on salads or drizzled over toast.

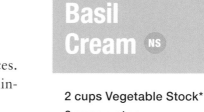
1. Fill a high-sided skillet with stock, water, and lemon slices. Bring to a simmer and add salmon. Cover and cook 12 to 15 minutes.

2. While salmon cooks, bring a large pot of salted water to a boil. Cook pasta according to package instructions.

3. Combine all sauce ingredients in a food processor or blender and puree until smooth.

4. Drain pasta and toss with all but ¼ cup basil sauce. Top with salmon and drizzle with remaining sauce and spicy mustard, if desired.

5. Serve immediately.

*See Vegetable Stock NS recipe (page 221).

▶ SERVES 4

2 cups Vegetable Stock*
2 cups water
1 lemon, sliced
1½ pounds salmon
1 pound spelt pasta

basil cream:
2 cups spinach
1 cup basil
1 clove garlic, minced
1 cup navy beans, rinsed and drained
2 teaspoons lemon zest
½ cup Vegetable Stock*
Spicy mustard, for serving (optional)

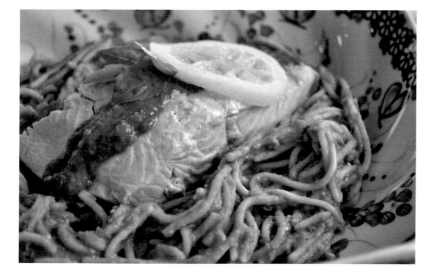

Salmon Soybean Cakes with Cilantro-Cream Sauce (NS)

1 pound wild salmon, cooked

1 cup cooked soybeans

1 teaspoon chopped scallions

1 teaspoon fresh rosemary

1 teaspoon fresh thyme

Sea salt, to taste

1 large egg, slightly beaten

½ cup bread crumbs*

2 teaspoons olive oil

sauce:

2 tablespoons walnuts

2 tablespoons olive oil

2 tablespoons hot water

¼ cup fresh cilantro

Sea salt, to taste

1. Flake cooked salmon into a bowl, being careful to remove any bones. Add beans, scallions, rosemary, thyme, and sea salt. Gently stir in egg and bread crumbs.

2. Form salmon mixture into baseball-size patties.

3. Heat olive oil in a large skillet over medium heat. Cook patties 3 to 4 minutes, turn, and cook an additional 3 to 4 minutes.

4. While the patties cook, blend walnuts in a food processor until a paste is formed. With food processor running, add olive oil and hot water, and process until creamy. Add cilantro and salt, and blend again until creamy and smooth.

5. Serve salmon cakes warm, and drizzle with cilantro-cream sauce.

*See Basic Bread Crumbs recipe (page 222).

▶ SERVES 4

Lemon-Ginger Salmon

1. Preheat oven to 400 degrees.

2. Rub 1 teaspoon olive oil on salmon and sprinkle with sea salt.

3. In a small bowl, mix lemon zest, lemon juice, remaining 1 teaspoon olive oil, ginger, and honey until combined. Brush evenly over the top of salmon.

4. Bake for 10 to 12 minutes.

5. Serve with Grilled Garlic-Ginger Bok Choy NS (page 133).

▶ SERVES 2

2 teaspoons olive oil, divided

1 pound wild salmon

½ teaspoon sea salt

Zest of 1 lemon

1 tablespoon lemon juice

2 tablespoons fresh ginger, peeled and grated

1 teaspoon honey (NS substitute agave)

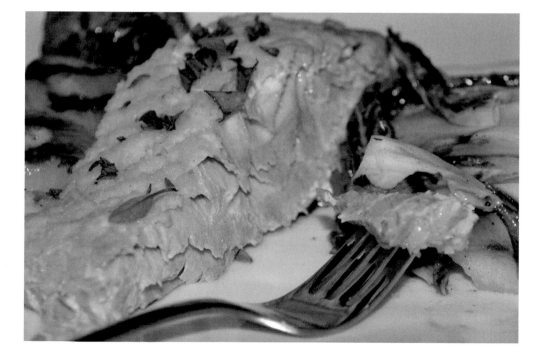

Baked Mahimahi with Fennel Salad (NS)

1 pound mahimahi

⅛ teaspoon ground coriander

1 teaspoon lemon zest

¼ teaspoon sea salt plus more to taste

fennel salad:

2 teaspoons chopped parsley

2 teaspoons olive oil

1 teaspoon lemon zest

2 teaspoons lemon juice

2 cups thinly sliced fennel

1 cup thinly sliced Granny Smith apples (NS substitute sliced plums)

1. Preheat oven to 350 degrees.

2. Season mahimahi with coriander, lemon zest, and ¼ teaspoon sea salt. Bake for 12 to 15 minutes, or until fish is flaky and white.

3. While the seafood bakes, whisk together parsley, olive oil, sea salt, to taste, lemon zest, and lemon juice in the bottom of a bowl. Add fennel and apple, and toss to combine.

4. Plate fish, top with fennel salad, and serve immediately.

▶ SERVES 2

tip: Don't rush when you have a sharp knife in your hand, no matter what the circumstance. Remember to tuck your fingers so your knuckles stick out slightly beyond the curl of your fingertips, so that the knife can glide harmlessly across your food, using your knuckles as a safety guide.

Parchment-Baked Snapper NS

1. Preheat oven to 375 degrees.

2. Cut 4 pieces of parchment paper into 12–15-inch sections. Fold parchment pieces in half and cut into a large heart shape, similar to cutting out a valentine. Place one snapper fillet in one half of the parchment heart, and season with salt, paprika, oregano, and garlic.

3. Top with peaches, tomatoes, and red onion, and drizzle each fillet with 1 teaspoon olive oil.

4. Fold edge of each parchment piece over; start at the top of the heart to roll and crease the edges. Crimp ends of parchment paper to seal the sides and place on a baking sheet. Bake for 12 to 15 minutes or until snapper is flaky and opaque and comes apart easily with a fork.

5. Serve warm.

▶ SERVES 2

1 pound (4 pieces) snapper fillets

½ teaspoon sea salt

½ teaspoon sweet paprika

1 tablespoon chopped fresh oregano

2 cloves garlic, minced

1 cup thinly sliced peaches

1 cup thinly sliced plum tomatoes

1 cup thinly sliced red onion

1 tablespoon olive oil, divided

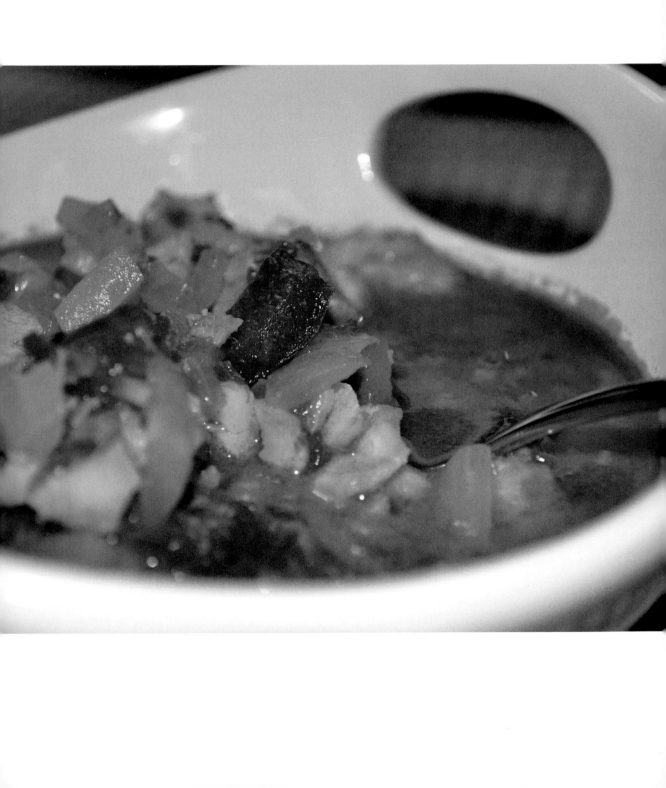

Spicy Seafood Stew

1. If using wakame, place in a bowl of cold water for 10 minutes.

2. Heat olive oil in a stockpot over medium heat. Sauté onion for 4 to 5 minutes. Add fennel, carrots and celery, and sauté an additional 3 to 4 minutes. Season with turmeric and fennel seeds, and add tomato paste and salt.

3. Drain wakame, rinse, and immediately add to stockpot.

4. Drain cans of pimiento, and pat dry. Puree in a food processor until very smooth. Add puree, bay leaves, and stock to stockpot. Let simmer 30 minutes.

5. While the stew simmers, dice cod and salmon into bite-size pieces. Add seafood to stockpot, and cook an additional 10 minutes or until seafood is cooked through.

6. Serve warm.

*See Vegetable Stock NS recipe (page 221).

▶ SERVES 4

¼ cup wakame (optional)
2 teaspoons olive oil
1 cup diced onions
1 bulb fennel, diced
1 cup diced carrots
½ cup diced celery
½ teaspoon turmeric
½ teaspoon fennel seeds
2 tablespoons tomato paste
Sea salt, to taste
2 (6½-oz.) cans pimiento
2 bay leaves
1 cup Vegetable Stock*
¾ pound cod
½ pound wild-caught salmon

featured ingredient

wakame

If you've had miso soup, you've most likely eaten wakame. Wakame is a nutrient-rich seaweed cultivated off the coast of Japan, and adds a briny finish to soups, stews, and even salads. It is most often dehydrated for distribution, but once soaked, returns to its dark-green color and velvety texture. Seaweed is a *Beneficial* food for Type AB, due to its abilities to detoxify the liver. Due to its mild flavor, wakame is a perfect way to begin adding seaweed to your diet.

 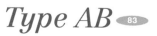

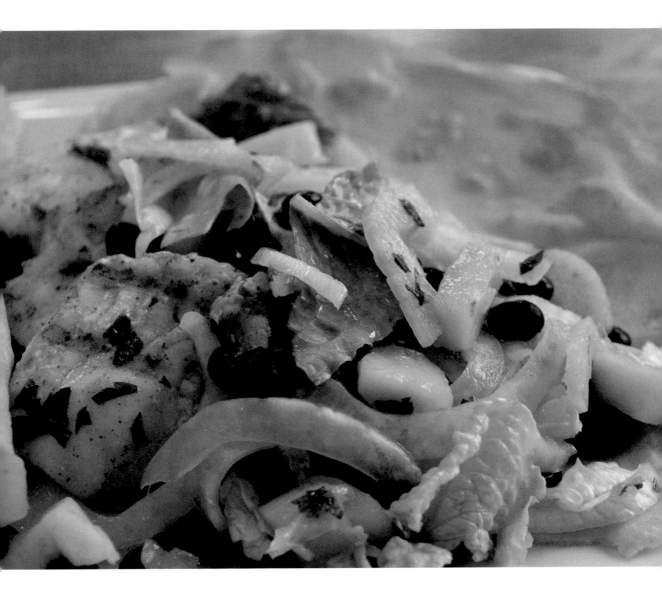

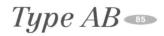
1. In a small bowl, combine chili powder, cumin, salt, paprika, and 1 tablespoon olive oil. Slice fish into 1-inch cubes and drizzle spice mixture over fish. Marinate in the refrigerator while preparing the rest of the dish, or at least 20 minutes.

2. Zest the lime, reserving ¼ teaspoon zest. Then, using a sharp knife, cut the ends off. Stand the lime on one end and slice off the sides, removing the skin and pith. Holding the lime over a bowl to capture the juices, cut between the membranes to remove the sections. Place lime sections and all remaining slaw ingredients in a large bowl, and toss to combine. Set aside while preparing rest of the dish to enable flavors to combine and textures to soften slightly.

3. Whisk all crêpe ingredients together in a large bowl. Heat a large skillet or crêpe pan over medium to medium-high heat and brush with ghee to create a nonstick surface. Using a ¼-cup measure, spoon crêpe batter into skillet, and quickly turn to spread batter into a very thin layer. Cook about 1 minute, or until the edges start to pull away from the skillet and tiny bubbles appear in the center of the crêpe. Using a large, flat spatula or carefully lifting edges with your hands, flip crêpe and cook 1 additional minute on the other side. Repeat with remaining batter. Stack crêpes on a plate and keep warm until serving.

4. Brush a heated grill pan with remaining 1 teaspoon olive oil and grill fish, 2 to 3 minutes per side, until fish is flaky and opaque.

5. To assemble tacos, place taco crêpe on a plate and top with fish and fennel slaw. Serve immediately.

▶ SERVES 4

¼ teaspoon chili powder

⅛ teaspoon cumin

½ teaspoon salt

¼ teaspoon paprika

1 tablespoon plus 1 teaspoon olive oil, divided

1 pound swordfish or other whitefish

fennel slaw:

1 thinly sliced fennel bulb

1 tablespoon chopped fresh mint

1 lime

2 teaspoons olive oil

½ cup diced pineapple

½ cup cooked pinto beans, drained and rinsed

¼ teaspoon sea salt

taco crêpe:

2 eggs

½ teaspoon sea salt

⅔ cup brown rice flour

2 tablespoons arrowroot starch

⅓ cup spelt flour

1 tablespoon olive oil

1½ cups (2 percent) cow's milk

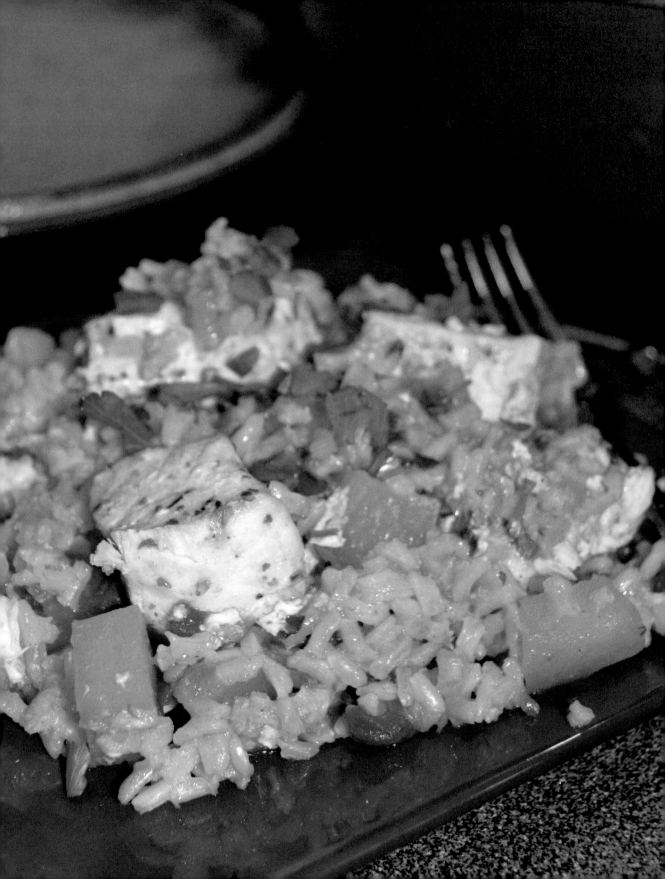

1. Preheat oven to 350 degrees.

2. In a large Dutch oven or paella pan, heat 1 teaspoon olive oil over medium heat. Sauté onion and sweet potato for 6 to 7 minutes, until onions become tender and potatoes start to soften. Add 1 teaspoon olive oil and add tomatoes, parsley, and garlic with the potatoes and onion. Sauté for 4 to 5 minutes, remove from pan, and set aside.

3. Add remaining 1 teaspoon olive oil to the same pan and toast brown rice for 2 minutes, stirring continuously. Rice will darken slightly in color and will start to give off a nutty smell. Add saffron, sea salt, paprika, and fresh oregano.

4. Return all vegetables to the Dutch oven with the rice, and stir to combine. Add stock, water and bay leaf. Bring to a simmer and cover. Place in oven and bake for 40 minutes.

5. While the paella cooks, dice seafood into 1-inch pieces, toss with dried oregano and sea salt, to taste.

6. Remove Dutch oven from oven, add seafood pieces, and bake an additional 12 minutes. Seafood should flake apart easily and rice will have absorbed all the liquid and become light and fluffy.

7. Serve warm.

*See Vegetable Stock NS recipe (page 221).

▶ SERVES 6

2 cups chopped yellow onion

1 cup sweet potato, peeled and cut into 1-inch dice

3 teaspoons olive oil, divided

2 vine-ripened tomatoes, chopped

¼ cup chopped parsley

2 teaspoons garlic, minced

1½ cups long-grain brown rice

15 threads saffron

1 teaspoon sea salt

½ teaspoon paprika

2 teaspoons fresh oregano, chopped

2 cups Vegetable Stock*

1 cup water

1 bay leaf

¾ pound tuna fillet

¾ pound red snapper fillet

1 teaspoon dried oregano

Seared Tuna with Fig and Basil Chutney (NS)

1 pound wild-caught tuna steaks

2 tablespoons plus 1 teaspoon olive oil

½ teaspoon sea salt

¼ cup fig jam

2 tablespoons chopped fresh basil

2 teaspoons lemon zest

2 tablespoons lemon juice

1. Drizzle tuna with 1 teaspoon olive oil and sprinkle both sides with sea salt.

2. In a small saucepan, whisk fig jam, basil, lemon zest, lemon juice, and remaining 2 tablespoons olive oil. Warm over low heat while tuna cooks.

3. Heat a skillet over medium heat and spray with nonstick olive oil cooking spray. Sear tuna for 1½ minutes per side. If you do not like your tuna rare inside, cook 2 to 3 minutes per side or until desired doneness.

4. Top tuna with fig and basil chutney and serve.

► SERVES 4

Roasted Turkey Breast NS

1. Preheat oven to 350 degrees.

2. Combine garlic, cumin, cinnamon, sea salt, and 2 teaspoons olive oil in a mini-chopper or food processor, and pulse until well combined. Spoon mixture over turkey breast, and massage into meat with your fingers.

3. In a large-bottomed skillet, heat remaining 1 teaspoon olive oil over medium heat. Add turkey and brown on each side, 3 minutes per side. Place turkey into a large baking dish and set aside.

4. In the same skillet used for turkey, add onions and carrots. Sauté about 5 minutes, and add sea salt, to taste.

5. Add tomato sauce, and stir to deglaze bottom of pan. Pour the carrots, onions, and tomato sauce around turkey in the baking dish. Add thyme and water so the liquid comes about three-quarters up the sides of the turkey breast. Cover with parchment paper and tinfoil (tinfoil does not react well with the acidity in tomatoes). Bake for 2 hours.

6. Remove from the oven, and place the baking dish over medium heat on the stovetop to thicken the tomato sauce.

7. Pull turkey meat apart with two forks, and plate with tomato sauce. Serve warm.

▶ SERVES 4

3 cloves garlic

1 teaspoon cumin

¼ teaspoon cinnamon

1 teaspoon sea salt

1 tablespoon olive oil, divided

1 (2–3 lb.) skinless turkey breast

1 red onion, chopped

2 white onions, chopped

3 large carrots, peeled and chopped

2 cups stewed tomato sauce

4 large sprigs fresh thyme

¾ cup water

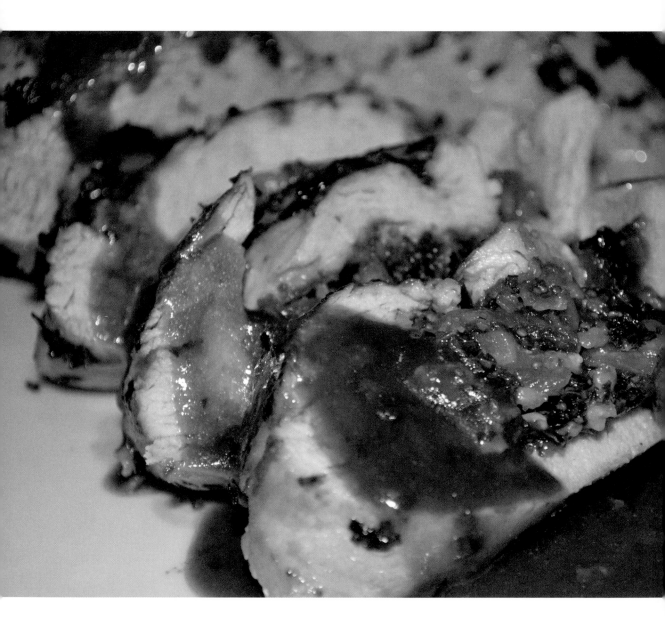

Herb-Crusted Turkey Breast Stuffed with Shallots and Figs NS

1. Preheat oven to 350 degrees.

2. Combine herbs in a small bowl. Set aside.

3. Heat 2 teaspoons olive oil and 1 teaspoon ghee in a skillet set over medium heat. Sauté shallots for 2 to 3 minutes. Add figs and kale, and sauté an additional 4 to 5 minutes. Remove from heat and toss with cheese.

4. Slice turkey breast in half to create two pieces. Butterfly breasts by placing on a cutting board and carefully slicing horizontally through the meat, leaving a ½-inch border. This opens the breast so that stuffing it is made simple. Divide kale stuffing evenly between turkey breasts. Gently pull the turkey back together and fasten with toothpicks. Sprinkle both sides of the stuffed turkey breasts with reserved herb mixture.

5. Heat remaining 1 teaspoon olive oil in an oven-safe skillet set over medium heat. Sear stuffed turkey breasts, 3 to 4 minutes per side. Transfer skillet to oven and bake in the oven for 8 to 10 minutes or until juices run clear and the internal temperature of the turkey reaches 165 degrees.

6. Remove turkey from pan and place on a cutting board to rest. In the meantime, place baking dish on the burner over medium heat and add remaining 1 tablespoon ghee and flour, whisking into a paste. Slowly add stock, whisking continuously to form a gravy. Bring to a simmer, and cook 2 to 3 minutes, until the gravy coats the back of a spoon.

7. Slice turkey breast and drizzle with gravy. Serve warm.

*See Turkey Stock NS recipe (page 220) or Vegetable Stock NS recipe (page 221).

▶ SERVES 4

Ingredients

1 tablespoons finely chopped oregano

2 tablespoons finely chopped thyme

2 tablespoons finely chopped basil

1 tablespoon olive oil, divided

1 teaspoon plus 1 tablespoon ghee, divided

½ cup shallots, minced

¾ cup chopped figs

2 cups chopped kale

½ cup soft goat cheese

1 large, boneless turkey breast

1 tablespoon brown rice flour

1 cup Turkey or Vegetable Stock*

Green Tea–Poached Turkey Tenderloin (NS)

4 cups water
8 green tea bags
1 pound turkey tenderloin
1 lemon, divided
½ teaspoon sea salt
1 cup fresh parsley
3 tablespoons olive oil
1 clove garlic
1 tablespoon water

1. In a high-sided skillet, bring water to a boil and steep the tea bags for 3 minutes. Reduce heat to medium and add turkey. Slice half the lemon and add to liquid with the sea salt. Cover and let cook 18 to 20 minutes or until the internal temperature of turkey reaches 165 degrees.

2. Puree parsley, olive oil, garlic, juice from the remaining half lemon, and water in a food processor until very smooth.

3. Serve turkey warm, topped with parsley oil.

▶ SERVES 4

1. Heat olive oil in a large pot over medium heat. Add onion and garlic, and sauté 4 to 5 minutes. Remove from heat and set aside.

2. In the same pot, brown turkey, breaking into bits with a flat spatula,6 to 8 minutes. Add onion mixture back to the pot along with remaining ingredients. Cover and let simmer at least 45 minutes. Stir occasionally to prevent burning.

3. Serve warm.

▶ SERVES 4

2 teaspoons olive oil

2 cups chopped yellow onion

1 clove garlic, minced

1 pound lean, ground turkey

8 tomatoes, diced

2 cups diced eggplant

¼ teaspoon cinnamon

1 teaspoon sea salt

2 teaspoons chili powder

1 teaspoon cumin

¼ cup tomato paste

1 (15-oz.) can navy beans, drained and rinsed

1 cup water

Turkey Pot Pie with Crunchy Topping

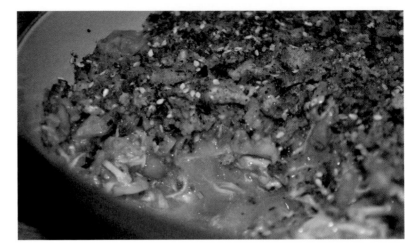

2 teaspoons olive oil

1 cup frozen pearl onions, thawed

1 cup carrots, diced

1 cup frozen sweet peas, thawed

1 cup fresh or frozen okra (thawed if frozen)

2 tablespoons oat flour

3¼ cups Turkey or Vegetable Stock*

1½ pounds roasted turkey breast, shredded*

¼ teaspoon saffron threads

½ teaspoon ground mustard

topping:

½ cup bread crumbs**

2 tablespoons sesame seeds

2 teaspoons ghee, melted

1 teaspoon olive oil

Spelt or whole-wheat store-bought crust (containing allowable grains)

1. Preheat oven to 375 degrees.

2. In a Dutch oven, heat olive oil over medium heat. Sauté onions, carrots, peas, and okra for 5 minutes. Sprinkle flour over vegetables and add broth, stirring to prevent lumps. Add roasted turkey, saffron, and ground mustard, stirring to combine. Cover and let cook 15 minutes, stirring occasionally.

3. Toss bread crumbs with sesame seeds, and drizzle with melted ghee and oil.

4. Uncover turkey filling, spoon into spelt crust, and top with bread crumb mixture. Place in the oven and bake 25 to 30 minutes, until crust is brown and turkey mixture is bubbling.

5. Serve warm.

*See Turkey Stock NS recipe (page 220) or Vegetable Stock NS recipe (page 221).

**See Basic Bread Crumbs recipe (page 222).

▶ SERVES 8

tip: I use leftover roasted turkey for this recipe, but if you're roasting from scratch, place a bone-in, skin-on turkey breast on a rack in a roasting pan. Rub with your favorite fresh-chopped herbs and bake at 350 degrees for 1½ to 2 hours until the internal temperature of turkey reaches 165 degrees.

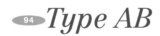

Turkey Meat Loaf

1. Preheat oven to 350 degrees. Line a baking sheet with parchment paper and set aside.

2. Place ground turkey in a large bowl and add all other ingredients. Use your hands to gently combine, being sure to not overwork the mixture.

3. Form meat into a large ball and place on prepared baking sheet. Shape turkey mixture into a log shape, about the length of the baking sheet and 3 to 4 inches thick. Bake in the oven for 45 minutes, until internal temperature of turkey reaches 165 degrees.

4. Serve warm.

*See Basic Bread Crumbs recipe (page 222).

▶ SERVES 4

1 pound ground turkey

1 cup diced onion

¼ cup finely diced carrot

¼ cup tomato paste

½ teaspoon mustard powder

1 clove garlic, minced

1 teaspoon paprika

1 large egg, lightly beaten

¾ cup bread crumbs*

 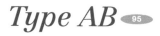

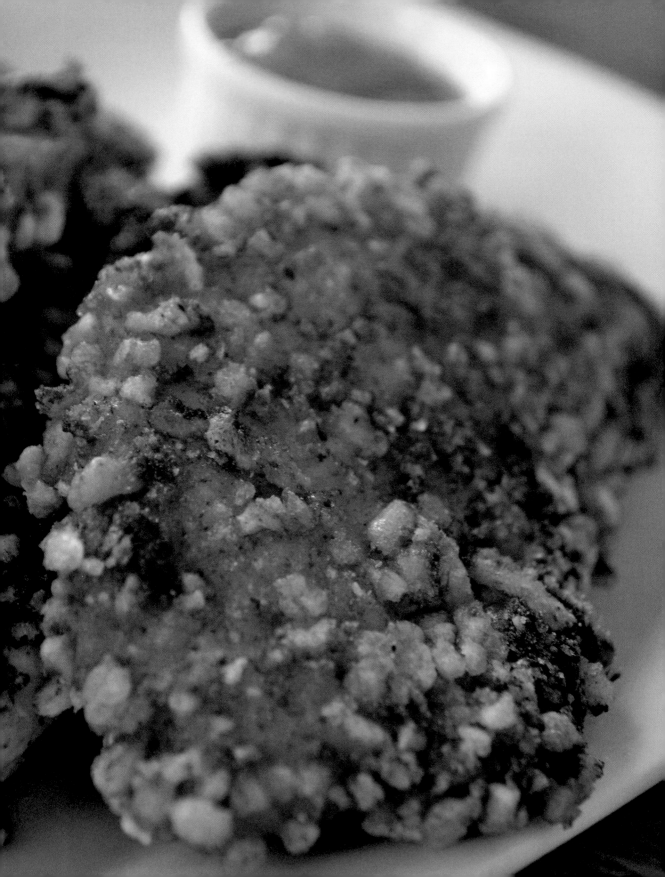

1. Grind rice cakes in a food processor or mini chopper until small crumbs form. Pour in a shallow bowl, add paprika and salt, and toss to combine.

2. In a separate, shallow bowl, whisk egg and milk. Dip tenderloins in egg mixture and then into rice cake mixture, being sure to coat each side.

3. Preheat oven to 375 degrees. Grease a baking sheet with non-stick spray and set aside.

4. Heat olive oil in a large, oven-safe skillet over medium heat, and brown tenderloins, about 5 minutes per side. Place onto prepared baking sheet and bake until cooked through, about 8 minutes or until the internal temperature reaches 165 degrees.

5. While the turkey cooks, whisk together all dipping sauce ingredients.

6. Serve warm.

▶ SERVES 4

tip: If you do not have an oven-safe skillet, simply wrap plastic handle tightly with tinfoil.

2 rice cakes

1 teaspoon sweet paprika

½ teaspoon sea salt

1 large egg

2 teaspoons (2 percent) cow's or goat's milk

4 turkey tenderloins

1 tablespoon olive oil

dipping sauce:

2 teaspoons ground mustard

2 tablespoons no sugar added apricot spread

1 teaspoon lemon juice

Broccolini-Stuffed Turkey Tenderloin

2 teaspoons ghee

1 bunch broccolini, roughly chopped

½ red onion, diced

Sea salt, to taste

¼ cup walnuts

⅓ cup crumbled feta cheese

1 cup Vegetable Stock*, divided

1 (1-lb.) turkey tenderloin

1 tablespoon olive oil

1 tablespoon brown rice flour

1 tablespoon oregano

1 tablespoon lemon juice

1. Preheat oven to 350 degrees.

2. Melt ghee in a large skillet over medium heat. Sauté broccolini and red onion in ghee until slightly tender, about 2 to 3 minutes. Remove from heat and season with salt to taste.

3. Combine broccolini and onions with walnuts, cheese, and ¼ cup stock in a food processor, and pulse to combine. Filling should be thick and pasty, similar in consistency to cookie dough. If mixture looks dry, add stock, 1 tablespoon at a time, to reach desired consistency. Set aside.

4. Butterfly the turkey tenderloin by positioning the tenderloin with the tip facing you and the thickest part of the meat facing your slicing hand. Put your hand on top of the tenderloin and insert the knife into the thickest part of the meat, carefully cutting across the tenderloin almost until you reach the opposite side. This will create a pocket for the filling.

featured ingredient

broccolini

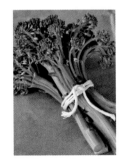

Broccolini looks like an elongated and tender version of broccoli. Broccolini has a slightly more mild taste, however, and is much more palatable when sautéed, roasted, or grilled. If cooked simply, it pairs best with olive oil and garlic. Broccolini is often confused with rappini or broccoli rabe, which has a much more bitter taste and is less appealing to most people.

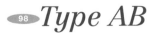

5. Spoon broccolini stuffing into center and secure the meat closed with toothpicks or cooking twine. Season outside of tenderloin with sea salt.

6. Heat olive oil in an oven-safe skillet set over medium heat. Brown tenderloin on both sides, about 2 minutes per side. Cover and place in oven for 20 to 25 minutes. Turkey is done when juices run clear and the internal temperature reaches 165 degrees.

7. Remove from oven, place turkey on a cutting board to rest, and place skillet back on stovetop. Add flour and gradually whisk in remaining stock, oregano, and lemon juice. Bring to a simmer and cook until thickened, 8 to 10 minutes. Season with sea salt, to taste, and serve over turkey.

*See Vegetable Stock NS recipe (page 221).

▶ SERVES 4

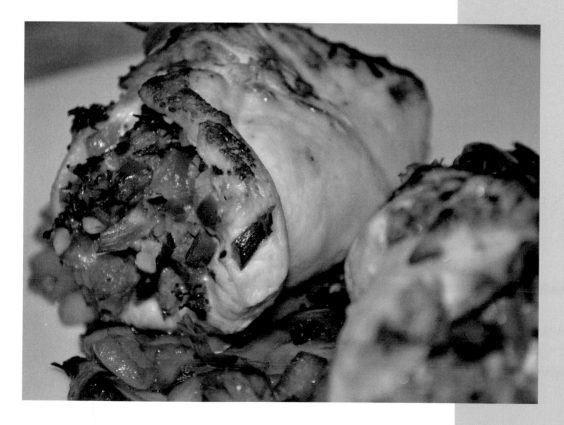

Turkey Sausage–Zucchini Boats

4 large zucchinis

2 tablespoons olive oil, divided

1 teaspoon fennel seeds

2 cloves garlic

¼ teaspoon mustard powder

1 cup diced onion

1 bulb fennel, diced

1 pound lean, ground turkey

1 tablespoon fresh thyme

2 tablespoons oat flour

1¼ cups chicken broth

1 (6½-oz.) can pimiento, drained

1 cup bread crumbs*

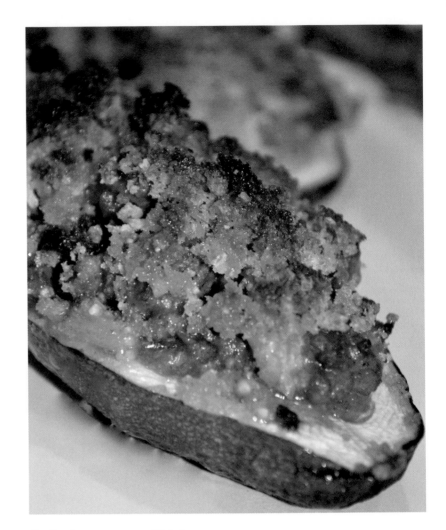

1. Preheat oven to 400 degrees.

2. Slice zucchini in half lengthwise. Use a spoon to scoop out the seeds, trying not to dig too deep into the flesh of the zucchini. Set zucchini skin side down on a baking sheet, drizzle with 2 teaspoons olive oil, and bake for 20 minutes.

3. Heat 2 teaspoons olive oil in a large skillet over medium heat. Add fennel seeds, garlic, and mustard powder and heat for 30 seconds, just to bring out the flavors. Add onion and fennel, and sauté 4 minutes. Add ground turkey, breaking large pieces apart with a flat wooden spoon, and cook until browned, 6-8 minutes.

EAT RIGHT FOR YOUR TYPE PERSONALIZED COOKBOOK

4. Once crumbled, add thyme and sprinkle with flour, tossing to coat. Slowly pour chicken broth over the turkey mixture, stirring constantly. Flour mixture will thicken to create a sauce. Bring sauce to a simmer then reduce heat to low.

5. Puree pimiento in a mini-chopper and add to skillet. Cook 5 to 6 minutes or until turkey is cooked through.

6. Remove zucchini from the oven. Spoon turkey mixture evenly into each roasted zucchini half, top with bread crumbs, and drizzle 1 teaspoon olive oil over each. Place zucchini back into the oven and bake 12 minutes or until steaming hot and bread crumbs are golden brown.

*See Basic Bread Crumbs recipe (page 222).

▶ SERVES 4

Shredded Turkey Bake NS

3 teaspoons olive oil, divided

1 cup diced carrots

1 cup diced onion

1 cup cauliflower florets

1 (1½-lb.) turkey tenderloin

1½ tablespoons fresh thyme, divided

2 cups carrot juice

1 cup Vegetable Stock*

Sea salt, to taste

1 tablespoon arrowroot starch

2 tablespoons cold water

½ cup quinoa

1 cup bread crumbs*

¼ cup shredded mozzarella cheese

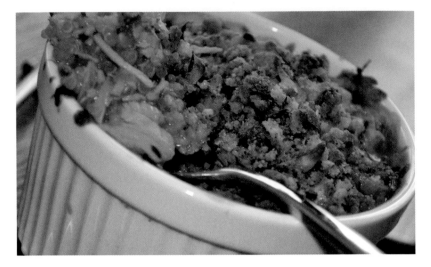

1. Heat 2 teaspoons olive oil in a large Dutch oven over medium heat. Add carrots and onion and sauté for 2 to 3 minutes. Add cauliflower and sauté an additional 5 minutes. Add turkey, 1 tablespoon thyme, carrot juice, stock, and salt, to taste. Bring to a boil, cover, reduce heat, and keep at a low simmer for one hour.

2. After one hour, uncover, remove turkey to a cutting board, and shred into bite-size pieces. Return turkey to the pot and increase the heat to medium to reduce carrot juice. In a small bowl, dissolve arrowroot starch in water. Add to shredded turkey mixture, stir to help the liquid thicken, and cook 10 minutes.

3. Add quinoa and cook an additional 12 minutes.

4. Preheat oven to 375 degrees.

5. Combine bread crumbs with remaining 1 teaspoon olive oil, ⅛ teaspoon salt, and remaining 1 teaspoon fresh thyme. Toss with cheese.

6. Spoon turkey mixture into 6 (7-oz.) ramekins, top with bread crumb mixture, and bake for 8 to 10 minutes or until turkey mixture is bubbling and topping is melted.

*See Vegetable Stock NS recipe (page 221). See Basic Bread Crumbs recipe (page 222).

▶ SERVES 6

EAT RIGHT FOR YOUR TYPE PERSONALIZED COOKBOOK

Hearty Slow-Cooker Turkey Stew NS

1. Preheat slow cooker to medium.

2. Heat olive oil in a large skillet over medium heat, and brown turkey breast on all sides. Remove from pan and set aside.

3. In the same skillet, add onion and parsnips and sauté 3 to 4 minutes. Add vegetables to the bottom of the slow cooker. Place turkey breast on top of vegetables and top with rosemary and thyme.

4. Pour water and stock in the bottom of the skillet to deglaze, scraping up all the bits. Pour liquid and bits over turkey in the slow cooker and cover.

5. Let cook 1 hour, then add the kale and cook 1 additional hour.

6. Serve warm.

*See Vegetable Stock NS recipe (page 221).

▶ SERVES 4

1 pound turkey breast
2 teaspoons olive oil
2 cups diced onion
2 cups diced parsnips
2 large sprigs fresh rosemary
4 large sprigs fresh thyme
1 cup water
1 cup Vegetable Stock*
4 cups red kale, torn

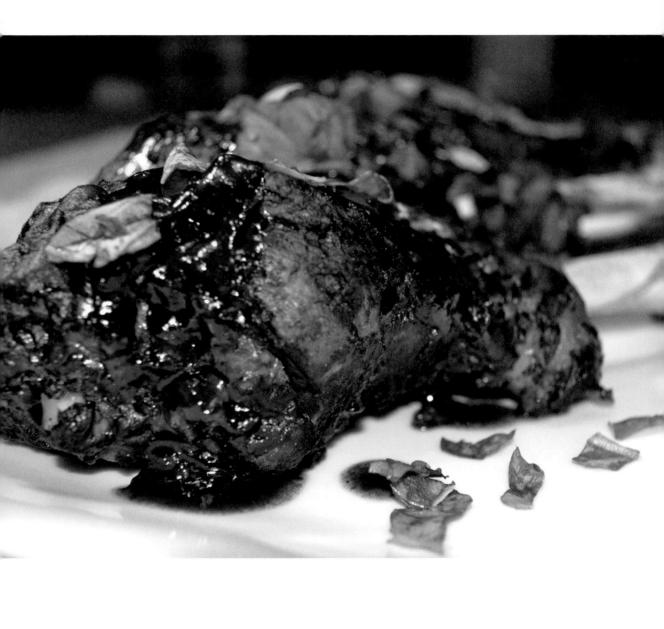

Turkey Mole Drumsticks

1. Preheat oven to 325 degrees.

2. Heat ghee in a medium skillet over medium heat. Sauté garlic and onion for 4 to 5 minutes, until tender and slightly browned. Add cumin, sea salt, chili powder, and cinnamon. Stir to combine and cook an additional 2 minutes. Add tomatoes, stock and peanut butter, stir to combine, and cook 3 to 4 minutes.

3. Remove from heat, stir in chocolate and transfer to a food processor. Puree mixture until smooth. As an optional step, push mole sauce through a strainer to have a silky-smooth sauce.

4. Reserve one-third of sauce. Remove skin from turkey drumsticks and coat with remaining mole sauce. Place in a baking dish, cover and bake for 1 to 1 ½ hours, until internal temperature of turkey reaches 165 degrees.

5. Warm reserved mole sauce in a small saucepan over medium heat. Serve turkey warm, topped with mole sauce.

*See Vegetable Stock NS recipe (page 221).

▶ SERVES 2

1 teaspoon ghee

2 cloves garlic, minced

¼ cup diced onion

1 teaspoon ground cumin

1 teaspoon sea salt

2 teaspoons ancho chili powder

½ teaspoon ground cinnamon

1½ cups diced vine-ripened tomatocs

¼ cup Vegetable Stock*

2 teaspoons peanut butter

1 ounce 100 percent dark chocolate, shaved

Turkey drumsticks

Lamb Steaks in Wild-Mushroom Sauce (NS)

1 teaspoon paprika

½ teaspoon sea salt

1 teaspoon dried thyme

1 pound lamb steak

3 teaspoons olive oil, divided

1 teaspoon ghee

1 cup diced onions

8 ounces cremini mushrooms, diced

2 cups diced maitake mushrooms

1 tablespoon fresh thyme

1. Combine paprika, sea salt, and dried thyme in a small bowl, and set aside.

2. Dice lamb steak into 2-inch pieces. Sprinkle spices evenly over the lamb, rubbing in with your hands to evenly distribute.

3. Heat 2 teaspoons olive oil in a large sauté pan over medium heat, and sear lamb, 3 minutes per side. The lamb will be browned and crispy while the center remains light pink. Remove from pan and set aside.

4. In the same skillet, add remaining olive oil, ghee, and onion. Sauté 3 to 4 minutes, add mushrooms and fresh thyme, and sauté an additional 8 to 10 minutes. Return lamb to the pan and toss to combine.

5. Serve hot.

▶ SERVES 4

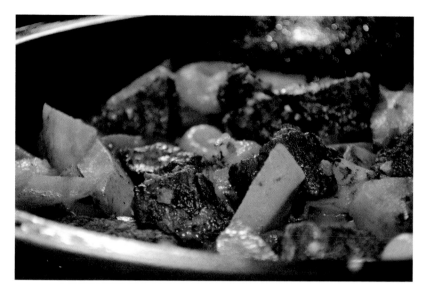

Moroccan Lamb Tagine

2 teaspoons minced garlic

2 teaspoons minced ginger

¼ teaspoon ground cinnamon

¼ teaspoon ground cumin

½ teaspoon turmeric

8 ounces lamb fillets

2 teaspoons olive oil, divided

10 cipollini onions, peeled

1 cup chopped carrots

1 cup chopped parsnips

½ cup Vegetable Stock*

1 tablespoon lemon juice

1. In a small bowl, combine garlic, ginger, cinnamon, cumin, and turmeric. Rub spices on lamb fillets. Heat tagine over medium-high heat, and brush with 1 teaspoon olive oil. When the tagine is hot, sear lamb in tagine just until browned on both sides, 1 to 2 minutes per side. Remove lamb and set aside.

2. Add remaining olive oil, onions, carrots, and parsnips to the tagine, and cook 5 to 6 minutes.

3. Reduce heat to low. Place pieces of lamb on top of vegetables, and add stock and lemon juice. Cover and let cook for 1½ hours.

4. Uncover and serve warm. Most of the liquid should be absorbed, and lamb and vegetables will be tender.

*See Vegetable Stock NS recipe (page 221).

▶ SERVES 4

tip: A tagine is a Moroccan cooking vessel that has a heavy, cast iron or clay base and a domed, pyramid-shaped top, which creates a slow-cooking method that adds moisture to each dish. As an alternative, try a cast iron skillet and cover tightly with tented tinfoil to create a seal.

Sweet Potato Shepherd's Pie (NS)

2½ teaspoons olive oil, divided

3 cloves garlic, divided

2 medium sweet potatoes, about 4 cups

1 tablespoon chopped fresh sage

1 tablespoon ghee, divided

6 tablespoons (2 percent) cow's or goat's milk

Sea salt, to taste

1 pound ground beef

2 teaspoons paprika

2 tablespoons brown rice flour

1½ cups beef broth

2 cups pearl onions*

1 cup peas

2 cups finely diced carrots

1 cup mozzarella cheese

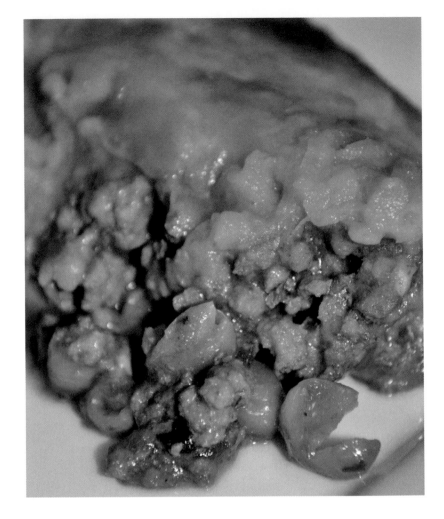

1. Preheat oven to 375 degrees.

2. Drizzle ½ teaspoon olive oil over 2 cloves of garlic and season with sea salt. Wrap garlic in parchment paper and then tinfoil, and roast in the oven for 25 minutes.

3. While the garlic roasts, peel and dice sweet potatoes into 2-inch pieces and place in a stockpot with enough water to cover. Bring to a boil and cook 12 to 15 minutes, just until easily pierced with a fork. Drain and transfer back into the empty pot or a clean bowl. Using a hand mixer, beat sweet potatoes with roasted garlic, sage, ghee, and milk. Season with sea salt, to taste, and set aside.

4. Reduce oven temperature to 350 degrees.

5. Heat remaining olive oil in a large skillet over medium heat. Brown ground beef, breaking up using a flat-ended spatula, 5 to 6 minutes. Add paprika and flour, stirring to coat. Mince remaining clove of garlic and add to skillet with beef broth. Bring the mixture to a simmer, reduce heat to low, and cook for 5 minutes.

6. Add onions, peas, and carrots to beef mixture and stir to combine. Pour into a 9" × 11" baking dish, top with sweet potato mixture, spreading evenly across the top with an offset spatula. Sprinkle cheese evenly over top and bake for 30 to 35 minutes, until mixture is bubbling and cheese is melted and slightly browned. Serve warm.

► SERVES 6

tip: Frozen pearl onions can be substituted in this recipe as a time-saver.

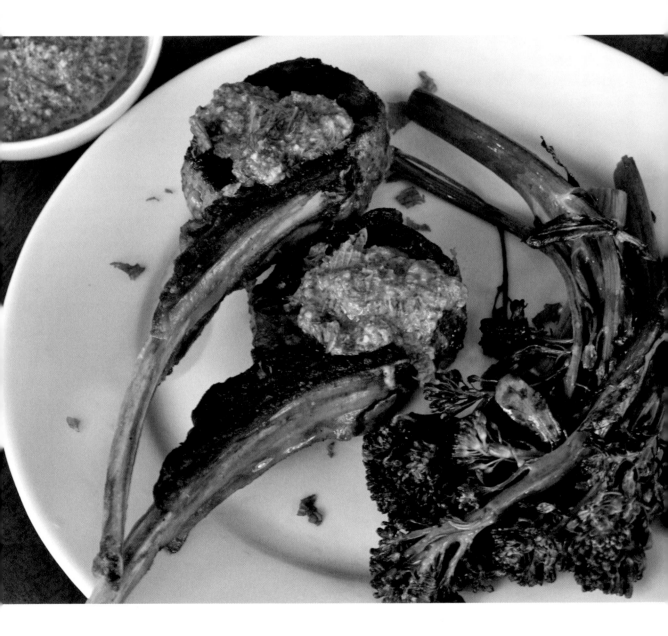

Grilled Lamb Chops with Mint Pesto (NS)

1. Season lamb with salt, place in a sealable glass container, and toss with ½ cup olive oil and garlic. Refrigerate at least an hour. Remove from fridge, and let come to room temperature.

2. Combine all pesto ingredients in a food processor and pulse until smooth. Spoon into a small bowl and set aside.

3. Heat a grill pan over medium, and brush with olive oil. Grill lamb 6 to 7 minutes on each side for medium doneness.

4. Top with pesto, and serve with Forbidden Black Rice Risotto (page 157).

▶ SERVES 4

1 pound French-rib lamb chops

Sea salt, to taste

½ cup olive oil plus more for grilling

3 cloves garlic, chopped

pesto:

½ cup fresh spinach

1 bunch fresh mint

1 teaspoon minced garlic

¼ cup extra virgin olive oil

½ teaspoon sea salt

Juice of 1 lemon

¼ cup raw walnuts

Red Quinoa–Mushroom Casserole (NS)

1 cup red quinoa

2 cups water

3 teaspoons ghee, divided

1 cup diced maitake mushrooms

1½ cups diced zucchini

½ cup finely diced shallots

½ teaspoon mustard powder

½ teaspoon dried ginger

2 cloves garlic, minced

2 tablespoons fresh oregano

¾ cup finely diced pineapple

1 cup Vegetable Stock*

5 large eggs, divided

1. Preheat oven to 350 degrees. Grease a 9" × 11" baking dish with nonstick olive oil cooking spray and set aside.

2. Combine quinoa and water in a saucepan and bring to a boil. Reduce heat and simmer for 12 minutes. Remove from heat and fluff with a fork.

3. Melt 2 teaspoons ghee in a large skillet over medium heat. Add mushrooms, zucchini, and shallots, and sauté 6 to 7 minutes, until vegetables are slightly tender. Remove from heat and set aside.

4. In a small bowl, whisk mustard powder, ginger, garlic, oregano, pineapple, stock, and 3 eggs.

5. Toss quinoa with mushroom mixture and place in prepared baking dish. Pour egg mixture evenly over casserole, using a fork to make sure the liquid reaches all corners of the casserole. Bake for 35 minutes.

6. Just before removing casserole, fry remaining eggs in a skillet with 1 teaspoon ghee and serve on top of casserole. Serve warm.

*See Vegetable Stock NS recipe (page 221).

▶ SERVES 6

featured ingredient

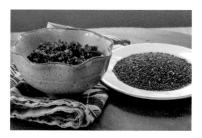

red quinoa

Red quinoa is almost identical in nutritional content to regular quinoa, and is a terrific source of fiber and protein, as it contains all nine essential amino acids. It also has a similar texture—light and fluffy with a slight crunch—to regular quinoa. The difference is that red quinoa has an earthier and less bitter taste. Use red quinoa in savory recipes, adding hearty vegetables, allowable cheeses, or beans.

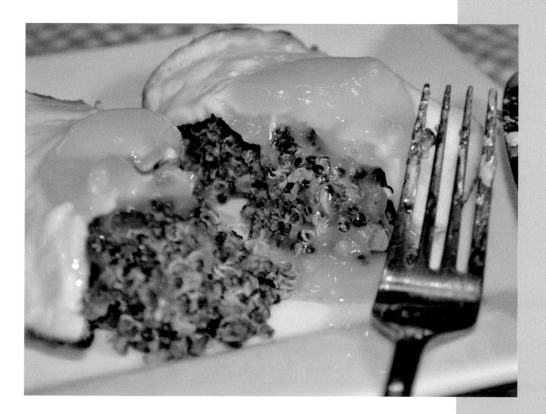

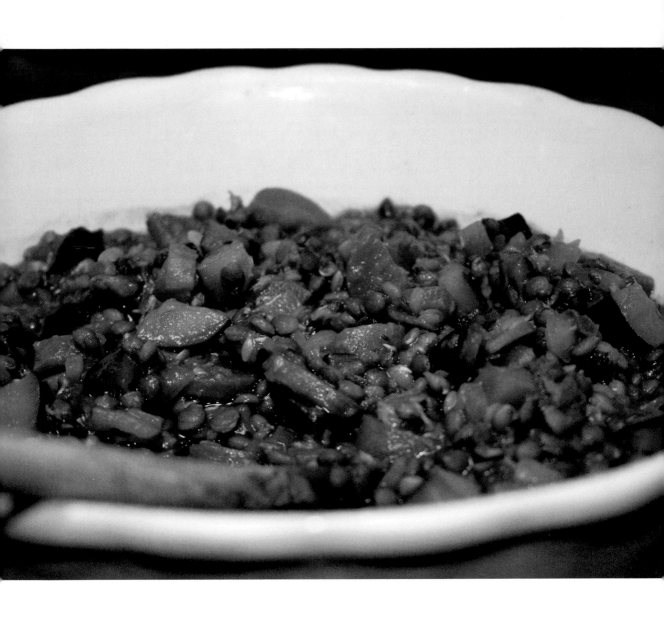

1. Place sprouted lentils in a bowl and cover with warm water. Soak for 25 minutes, then drain.

2. Heat olive oil in a large Dutch oven set over medium heat. Add onion, carrots, parsnips, zucchini, and cumin, and sauté 6 to 7 minutes. Add lentils and cook 1 additional minute.

3. Add stock, 1 cup at a time, stirring after each addition. Season with salt, to taste. Let cook an additional 30 minutes.

4. Serve warm.

*See Vegetable Stock NS recipe (page 221).

▶ SERVES 4

1 cup sprouted lentils
1 tablespoon olive oil
1 cup diced onions
¾ cup diced carrots
¾ cup diced parsnips
2 zucchini, diced
½ teaspoon cumin
5 cups Vegetable Stock*
Sea salt, to taste

featured ingredient

sprouted lentils

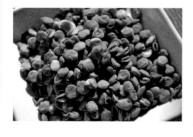

Anytime you see the word **sprouted** in connection with a grain, legume, or seed, it simply means that the food enzymes have been activated, which results in increased nutrient content. Sprouted lentils can be found at most natural foods stores, and cook up much faster than lentils that have not been sprouted, so they are a great addition to your "fast food" repertoire.

Slow-Cooker Butternut Squash– Lentil Stew NS

1 cup chopped onion

1 cup chopped carrots

1 tablespoon olive oil

1 pound green lentils

1 teaspoon sea salt

2 cups Vegetable Stock*

2 cups cubed butternut squash

¼ teaspoon cumin

1 teaspoon ground ginger

1 teaspoon garlic powder

¼ teaspoon cinnamon

1 tablespoon chopped fresh sage

3 cups water

1. Turn your slow cooker to high setting.

2. Add all ingredients to the slow cooker. Stir gently to evenly distribute spices and vegetables.

3. Cook 2½ to 3 hours. Stew should be thick and tender, and most of the liquid will be absorbed.

4. Serve warm.

*See Vegetable Stock NS recipe (page 221).

▶ SERVES 4

Lentil Burgers

1. Place 1 cup of lentils in a large bowl and smash using a fork or potato masher.

2. Add remaining 1 cup lentils, spinach, carrots, 1 tablespoon olive oil, thyme, sea salt, garlic, bread crumbs, and egg, mixing gently just to combine. Form into 6 patties and set aside on a plate.

3. Heat remaining 2 teaspoons olive oil in large skillet over medium heat. Cook burgers, about 4 minutes per side, until browned and crispy and warm in the center.

4. Serve warm with caramelized onions, sliced tomato, and crunchy lettuce on toasted sprouted wheat rolls.

*See Basic Bread Crumbs recipe (page 222).

▶ SERVES 4

2 cups cooked green lentils

1½ cups chopped spinach

½ cup carrot, shredded

1 tablespoon plus 2 teaspoons olive oil, divided

1 tablespoon fresh thyme

½ teaspoon sea salt

2 cloves garlic, minced

½ cup bread crumbs*

1 large egg, beaten

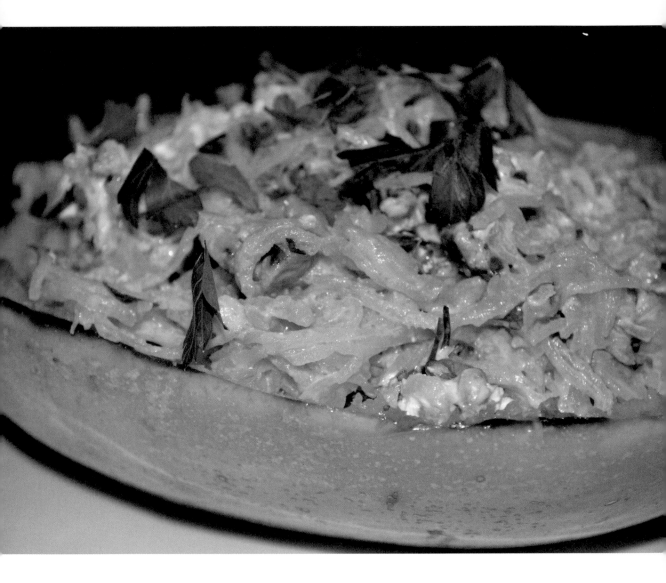

Spaghetti Squash with Creamy Goat Cheese, Walnut, and Parsley Sauce NS

1. Preheat oven to 350 degrees.

2. Carefully halve squash from stem to base and, using a metal spoon, scoop out seeds. Brush 2 teaspoons olive oil and sprinkle sea salt over flesh of squash. Roast cut side down on a baking sheet for 35 to 40 minutes. Squash should be browned on the skin, and flesh should be easily pierced with a fork.

3. While squash cooks, heat remaining 1 teaspoon olive oil in a small skillet over medium heat. Sauté onion for 4 to 5 minutes, or until tender. Remove from heat and add goat cheese, walnuts, and parsley.

4. Remove squash from oven and let cool 5 minutes. Take a fork and scrape insides of squash from stem to base. Spaghetti squash will peel away from the skin in long strings, resembling spaghetti. Place strands of squash into a large bowl and toss with goat cheese mixture.

5. Serve warm.

▶ SERVES 4

1 large spaghetti squash

1 tablespoon olive oil, divided

½ teaspoon sea salt

¼ cup very finely diced onion

3 ounces goat cheese

1 cup toasted diced walnuts

1 cup finely diced parsley

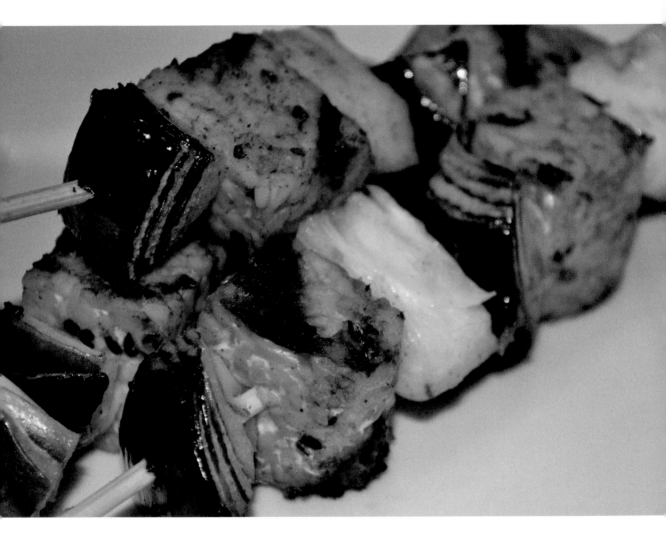

1. Soak 8 to 10 bamboo skewers in water for up to 1 hour before use to prevent burning.

2. Whisk lemon juice, agave, olive oil, ginger, paprika, and garlic in a bowl. Dice tempeh into 1-inch cubes and place in a glass storage dish with a sealable lid and pour ⅔ of the marinade over the tempeh, tossing to make sure all sides are coated with the marinade. Cover and place in the refrigerator for 3 hours.

3. Preheat grill or grill pan.

4. Begin skewering by alternating one piece of tempeh, pineapple, and onion twice on each skewer and brush pineapple and onion with marinade. Grill for 5 to 6 minutes, flipping halfway through cooking and brushing with any remaining marinade.

5. Serve warm.

▶ SERVES 4

2 tablespoons fresh lemon juice

1 tablespoon agave

3 tablespoons olive oil

1 tablespoon minced fresh ginger

½ teaspoon sweet paprika

1 teaspoon garlic, minced

1 (8-oz.) package organic flax tempeh

4 cups pineapple pieces

1 red onion, cut into ½-inch dice

featured ingredient

tempeh

Tempeh is fermented soybeans that are pressed into a ½-inch to 1-inch cake, providing a firm texture and slightly nutty taste. Widely used in Indonesia, tempeh has become popular among vegetarians in the United States. Like tofu, tempeh has the ability to absorb any flavor you choose to season it with, so it is a perfect canvas for your culinary genius. As a bonus, it is packed with protein and few calories, making it an ideal substitution for beef or any animal protein.

Ginger-Tofu Stir-Fry NS

8 ounces extra-firm tofu

3 teaspoons olive oil, divided

1 (2-inch) piece ginger, peeled and thinly sliced

2 cups snow peas

1 cup sliced bok choy

¼ cup bamboo shoots

⅓ cup plum jam

1 tablespoon lemon juice

1 tablespoon lemon zest

1 tablespoon low-sodium soy sauce (made from soy)

1 tablespoon agave

1. Remove tofu from packaging and pat dry with a paper towel. Slice horizontally and place on another paper towel to dry each side. After about 10 minutes, dice tofu into 1-inch cubes.

2. In a large wok or sauté pan, heat 2 teaspoons olive oil over medium heat. Add ginger and sauté 1 minute. Add tofu and stir-fry until browned, about 3 to 4 minutes. Remove from wok and set aside.

3. Add remaining 1 teaspoon olive oil, snow peas, bok choy, and bamboo shoots, and stir-fry 3 to 4 minutes. Add tofu back to the wok along with remaining ingredients. Toss to coat and cook 2 minutes.

4. Serve hot.

▶ SERVES 4

tip: Bamboo shoots are most commonly found in cans, in the ethnic aisle at the grocery store or natural food market. Rinse bamboo shoots and pat dry so they are ready for cooking.

Soups and Sides

Many times when preparing dinner, we think about eating a protein, vegetable, and complex carbohydrate, and although having them all together in one pot like chili or lasagna is ideal, it doesn't always work out that way. Therefore, it is essential to have a collection of quick and delicious side or soup options to pair with your protein choice. A number of vegetables or complex carbohydrate–based soups and sides can be found in this section.

Thai Curry Soup (NS)

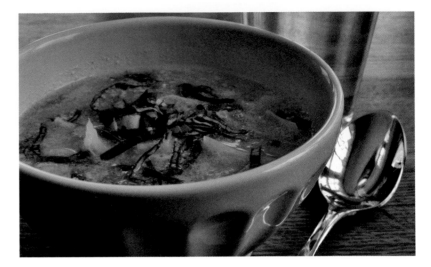

2–3 teaspoons olive oil

1 cup diced onion

1 teaspoon garlic, minced

1 tablespoon ginger, minced

⅛ teaspoon turmeric

¼ teaspoon curry powder

1 cup diced celery

Sea salt, to taste

2 small turnips, diced

1 lemongrass stick

4 cups water

cream sauce:

¼ cup thick yogurt

1 teaspoon agave

1. Heat olive oil in a stockpot over medium heat. Sauté onion, garlic, and ginger for 3 to 4 minutes, until slightly tender and aromatic. Add turmeric, curry powder, celery, sea salt, and turnips, stir, and cook 5 minutes.

2. Bruise lemongrass by hitting the stalk several times with the back of your knife, to bring out the flavors.

3. Add water to the stockpot. Add lemongrass, cover, and simmer at least 30 minutes.

4. While the soup simmers, prepare the cream sauce by stirring yogurt with agave, set aside.

5. Remove lemongrass from soup just before serving. Serve warm with a dollop of yogurt cream sauce.

▶ SERVES 6

featured ingredient

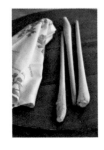

lemongrass

Lemongrass is a thick, woody stalk that needs to be bruised and chopped before use, to help bring out its flavor. Lemongrass is most widely used in Asian cooking, and adds a fresh, citrus flavor to dishes. Add to soups, rice, or quinoa for a great, new twist on an ordinary recipe.

EAT RIGHT FOR YOUR TYPE PERSONALIZED COOKBOOK

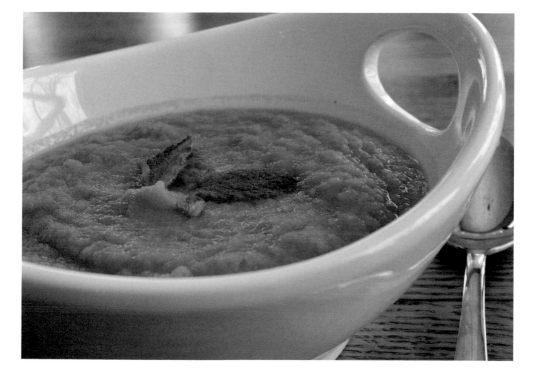
1. Heat olive oil and ghee in a large stockpot over medium heat. Add onion, garlic, and carrots, and sauté 5 to 6 minutes until vegetables become tender. Add remaining ingredients and bring to a boil, then reduce to a simmer, cover and cook at least 30 minutes, or until carrots are fork-tender.

2. Puree soup with an immersion blender or in batches in a standing blender until smooth. If the mixture is too thick, add water to reach desired consistency, about the thickness of cake batter.

3. Serve warm.

▶ SERVES 6

1 teaspoon olive oil

2 teaspoons ghee

1 cup chopped onion

1 clove garlic

2 pounds carrots, peeled and diced

1 (3-inch) piece ginger, peeled and grated (about ¼ cup)

½ teaspoon sea salt

1 tablespoon lemon zest

4 cups water

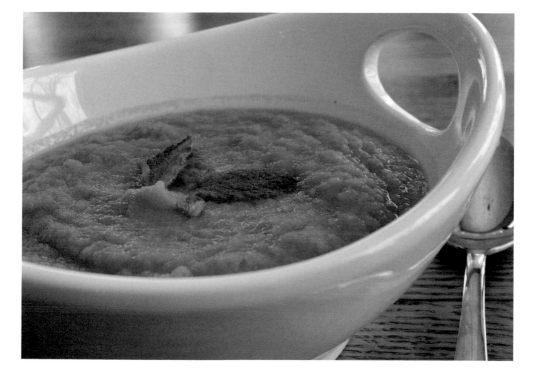

Roasted Parsnip Soup (NS)

4 cups diced parsnips

4 cups diced cauliflower

2 cloves garlic, peeled

2 tablespoons olive oil, divided

Sea salt, to taste

2 cups finely sliced sweet onion

2 Granny Smith apples, finely diced

1½ cups (2 percent) cow's or goat's milk

1 cup water

⅛ teaspoon nutmeg

¼ cup chopped fresh sage

1. Preheat oven to 375 degrees.

2. Place parsnips, cauliflower, and garlic on a sheet pan, drizzle with 1 tablespoon olive oil, and sprinkle with sea salt. Toss to coat.

3. Roast vegetables in the oven for 35 to 40 minutes, or until tender and golden brown around the edges.

4. About 15 minutes before the vegetables are finished cooking, heat remaining 1 tablespoon olive oil in a large stockpot over medium heat. Sauté onion for 8 to 10 minutes. Add apples and sauté an additional 3 to 4 minutes.

5. Add roasted vegetables and remaining ingredients to onion mixture. Bring the soup to a gentle boil and simmer for 20 minutes. Blend with an immersion blender or puree in batches in a standing blender. Season with additional sea salt, to taste, and serve warm.

▶ SERVES 6

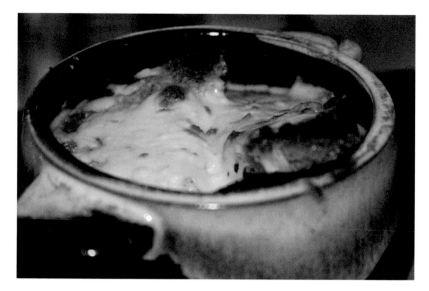

5 large white onions
1 tablespoon olive oil
½ tablespoon ghee
Sea salt, to taste
½ cup red or white wine
4 sprigs thyme
2 sprigs sage
2 bay leaves
3 cups Vegetable Stock*
4 slices sprouted bread
1 cup grated Gruyère cheese

1. Peel and slice onions in half and then slice into thin, half-moon shapes.

2. Heat olive oil and ghee in a large-bottomed stockpot over medium heat. Add onions and caramelize for 12 minutes. Season with sea salt, reduce temperature to medium-low, and cook an additional 20 minutes. Onions will become a rich caramel color as the natural sugars in the onions release and help sweeten them.

3. Add wine to the onions to deglaze the pan (help the delicious bits on the bottom of the pan come up and mingle with the onions) and cook 30 seconds. Add thyme, sage, bay leaves, salt, and stock. Simmer for 30 minutes.

4. Evenly divide soup among 4 (7-oz.) high-sided, oven-safe bowls or ramekins. Place 1 slice of bread on top of each ramekin, then sprinkle with cheese, to create a cheesy bread lid for the soup.

5. Broil in oven for 2 minutes or until the cheese begins to bubble and brown slightly. Keep a close eye on the broiler as the bread and cheese can burn quickly. Serve warm.

*See Vegetable Stock NS recipe (page 221).

▶ SERVES 4

Broccoli–Northern Bean Soup NS

1 tablespoon olive oil, divided

1 cup diced white onion

2 heads broccoli

1 clove garlic, minced

1 (15-oz.) can northern beans, rinsed and drained

2 cups Vegetable Stock*

4 sprigs fresh thyme

Sea salt, to taste

¼ cup pine nuts

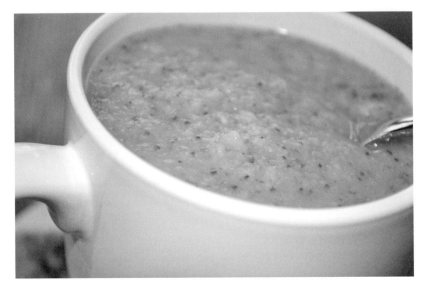

1. Heat 2 teaspoons olive oil in a large stockpot over medium heat. Add onion and sauté 5 to 6 minutes.

2. Trim woody stems off broccoli, and discard. Rough chop the broccoli and remaining stems. Add to the onions along with garlic, beans, stock, and thyme. Bring to a boil and reduce to simmer for 15 minutes. Vegetables should be fork-tender but not falling apart.

3. Puree with an immersion blender, or in batches in a stand blender. Soup should be thick and creamy but easily run off your spoon. Add water or additional stock if you prefer a thinner consistency. Season with sea salt, to taste.

4. Heat remaining 1 teaspoon olive oil in a small skillet set over low heat. Toast pine nuts for 2 to 3 minutes, or until golden brown.

5. Serve soup hot, topped with toasted pine nuts.

*See Vegetable Stock NS recipe (page 221).

▶ SERVES 6

EAT RIGHT FOR YOUR TYPE PERSONALIZED COOKBOOK

1. Heat 1 teaspoon olive oil in a Dutch oven set over medium heat. Sauté minced ginger and garlic, stirring continuously to prevent burning. Add remaining 1 teaspoon olive oil then toss in tofu, season with sea salt and cook until browned, about 1 to 2 minutes per side. Remove from pot and set aside.

2. Add stock, water, onions, carrots and bay leaf. Simmer over medium-low heat for 20 minutes.

3. Add beans and tofu mixture to the soup, and simmer 10 minutes. Spoon into bowls and top each with ½ cup escarole.

*See Vegetable Stock NS recipe (page 221).

▶ SERVES 4

2 teaspoons olive oil, divided

1 (1-inch) piece fresh ginger, peeled and minced

1 clove garlic, minced

12 ounces extra-firm tofu, cubed

Sea salt, to taste

2 cups Vegetable Stock*

3 cups water

1 cup pearl onions

1 bay leaf

1 cup carrots, matchsticks

2 cups haricot vert

2 cups shredded escarole

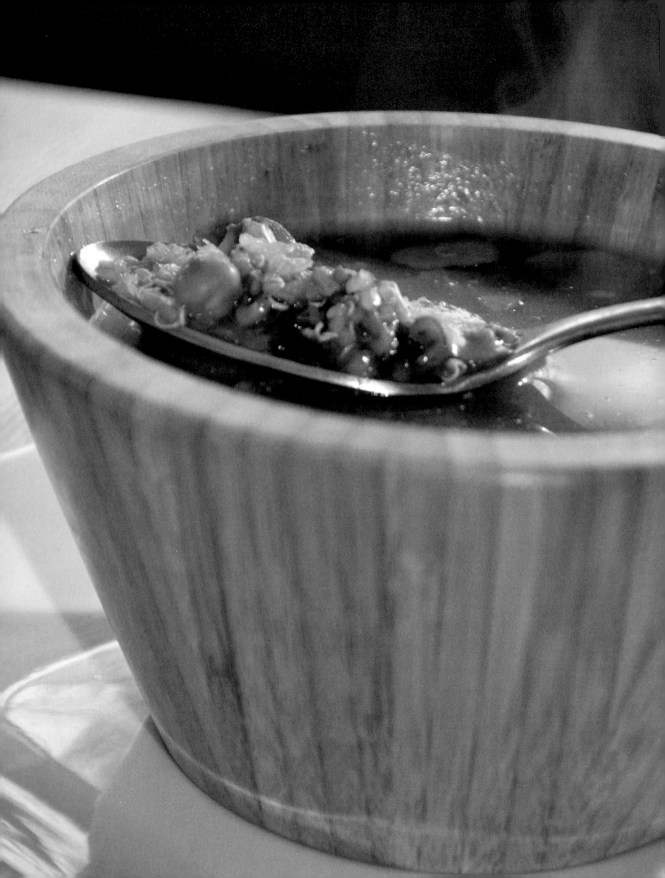

Wild-Grain Soup with Sun-Dried Tomato Pesto NS

1. Combine wild rice and 1 cup water in a stockpot, and cook according to package instructions. When rice is fluffy and has absorbed all the water, spoon into a separate bowl and set aside.

2. In the same pot, melt ghee over medium heat and add garlic, mushrooms, and celery. Sauté 3 to 4 minutes. Add stock and remaining 3 cups water. Bring to a boil, and reduce heat to a simmer, and cook 5 minutes.

3. Combine all pesto ingredients in a food processor and process until smooth and only small chunks remain. Season with sea salt, to taste.

4. Add quinoa to soup and simmer an additional 10 minutes. Add snow peas and cook 3 minutes. Divide soup evenly between bowls, and top each with a dollop of pesto.

*See Vegetable Stock NS recipe (page 221).

▶ SERVES 6

½ cup wild brown rice

4 cups water, divided

2 teaspoons ghee

1 clove garlic, minced

1 bunch maitake mushrooms, diced

½ cup diced celery

4 cups Vegetable Stock*

¼ cup quinoa

¾ cup snow peas

pesto:

½ cup sun-dried tomatoes (not in oil)

½ cup fresh basil

1 clove garlic

2 tablespoons olive oil

2 tablespoons lemon juice

¼ cup raw walnuts

3 tablespoons water

Broccoli and Cabbage Slaw

3 tablespoons lemon juice

3 tablespoons olive oil

2 teaspoons ground mustard

1 teaspoon honey or agave

Sea salt, to taste

2 cups red cabbage (about ½ small head)

2 cups broccoli stems (about 2 bunches)

½ cup golden raisins

¼ cup chopped parsley

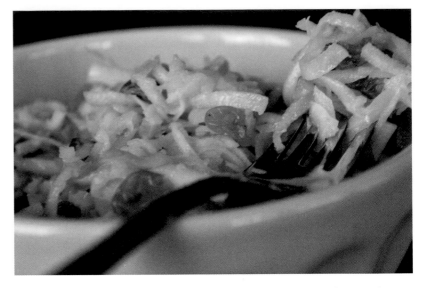

1. Whisk lemon juice, olive oil, mustard, honey, and sea salt in a large bowl, and set aside.

2. Remove tough bottoms from cabbage as well as the outer layers. Using a food processor or a hand grater, grate peeled cabbage, and add to the bowl with dressing. Cut bottoms and tops off broccoli stems, peel, and grate. Add broccoli to bowl.

3. Add raisins and parsley, and toss to combine vegetables with dressing. Serve chilled.

▶ SERVES 4

tip: Reserve broccoli tops for a fast and delicious side dish: mix with 2 teaspoons olive oil and a dash of sea salt, and roast in a 375-degree oven for 20 minutes.

EAT RIGHT FOR YOUR TYPE PERSONALIZED COOKBOOK

1. Heat grill pan over medium heat.

2. Pull the leaves off the base of the bok choy and slice off the very bottom of the stems to remove any tough pieces. Wash the leaves individually and let them dry completely on a kitchen towel.

3. In a small bowl, whisk olive oil, ginger, garlic, and agave. Brush individual bok choy leaves with ginger mixture. Grill leaves for about 30 to 45 seconds per side, so that leaves wilt and have golden-brown grill marks. Season with sea salt to taste.

4. Serve warm.

▶ SERVES 4

1 medium bunch bok choy

2 teaspoons olive oil

1 tablespoon fresh ginger, grated

1 clove garlic, minced

1 teaspoon agave

Sea salt, to taste

tip: When purchasing bok choy, look for stalks that are bright white in color with dark green leaves. Avoid spotted stems and wilted-looking leaves.

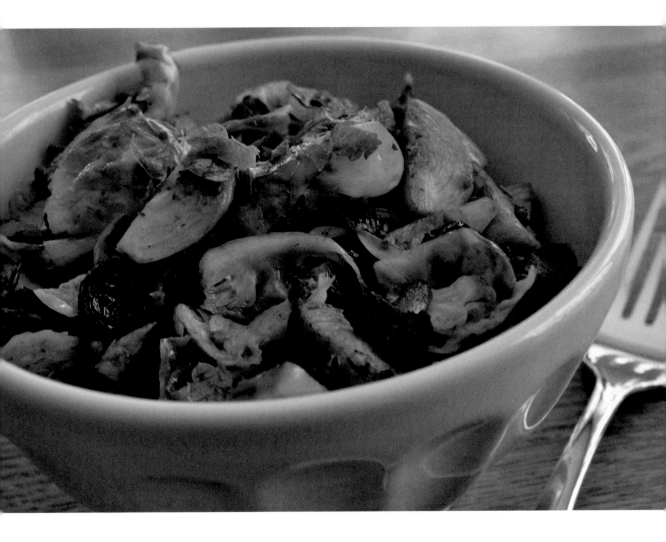

Sweet-and-Salty Brussels

1. Heat ghee and olive oil in a large skillet over medium heat. Sauté shallots and turkey bacon until bacon is crispy, about 4 to 5 minutes. Add Brussels sprouts and cook for 15 minutes, stirring occasionally to prevent burning. Add raisins and stock, stir to deglaze pan, and cook 3 minutes, until raisins become tender.

2. Sprouts are done when they can be pierced with a fork but still give moderate resistance. Be careful to avoid overcooking, as they can become mushy and lose a lot of flavor.

3. Garnish with parsley and serve warm.

*See Vegetable Stock NS recipe (page 221).

▶ **SERVES 4**

1 teaspoon ghee

2 teaspoons olive oil

2 tablespoons finely diced shallots

4 strips nitrate- / preservative-free turkey bacon, diced

4 cups quartered Brussels sprouts

¼ cup golden raisins

½ cup Vegetable Stock*

1 tablespoon chopped parsley, for garnish

South Indian–Curried Okra

1 tablespoon olive oil

½ teaspoon mustard seed

½ teaspoon cumin

½ teaspoon urad dal

¾ cup finely diced onion

3 cups diced okra

4 cups chopped spinach

½ teaspoon turmeric

½ teaspoon sea salt

1. Heat olive oil in a Dutch oven over medium heat. Add mustard seed, cumin, and urad dahl, and cook 30 seconds, stirring continuously to prevent burning. Add onion and cook 5 minutes.

2. Add okra and cook an additional 15 minutes.

3. Add spinach, turmeric, and salt, and cook 5 to 8 minutes, until okra is tender and spinach is wilted.

4. Serve warm.

▶ SERVES 6

Baked Beans

1. Preheat oven to 375 degrees.

2. Heat olive oil in a Dutch oven over medium heat. Sauté onion and garlic until translucent and tender, 5 to 7 minutes. Add mustard, molasses, salt, paprika, and chili powder, and cook 1 minute.

3. Add beans, tomato paste, and stock, and stir to combine.

4. Cover and bake for 25 minutes, until mixture is thick and warmed throughout. Serve warm.

*See Vegetable Stock NS recipe (page 221).

▶ SERVES 6

2 teaspoons olive oil

1 cup diced yellow onion

1 clove garlic, minced

1 teaspoon dry mustard

1 teaspoon molasses

1 teaspoon salt

1 teaspoon paprika

½ teaspoon chili powder

2 cans pinto beans, drained and rinsed

3 tablespoons tomato paste

⅓ cup Vegetable Stock*

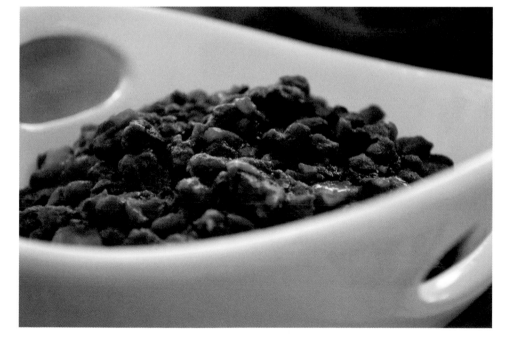

 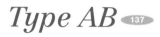

Spicy Collards

2 teaspoons olive oil

1 teaspoon ghee

½ cup diced shallots

4 slices nitrate- / preservative-free turkey bacon, finely diced

½ teaspoon chipotle chili powder

1 bunch collard greens

1 (15-oz.) can pinto beans, drained and rinsed

Sea salt, to taste

1. Heat olive oil and ghee in a large skillet over medium heat. Add shallots and bacon, and sauté until bacon is crispy, about 4 to 5 minutes.

2. Season with chili powder, add collard greens, and cook for 10 to 12 minutes, until collards are tender and partially wilted.

3. Add pinto beans and cook an additional 3 to 4 minutes, until warmed through.

4. Season with sea salt, to taste, and serve warm.

▶ SERVES 4

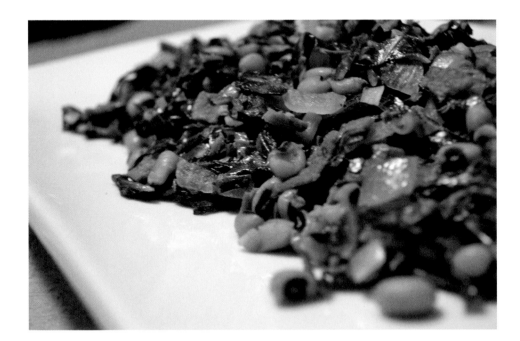

Garlic-Creamed Collards and Spinach NS

1. Heat olive oil in a Dutch oven over medium heat, and sauté garlic and onion for 2 to 3 minutes. Add collard greens and cook until wilted, about 5 to 6 minutes, season with sea salt, to taste. Remove from pan and set aside.

2. To the same pan, add oat flour, stir, and cook for 1 minute over medium heat to render out the taste of the flour. Slowly add milk and stock, stirring continuously to avoid lumps. Continue stirring until mixture becomes the consistency of yogurt, about 5 minutes.

3. Add spinach one-quarter at a time, allowing each batch to wilt before adding the next.

4. Once all the spinach has been added, serve warm.

*See Vegetable Stock NS recipe (page 221).

▶ SERVES 4

2 teaspoons olive oil

2 cloves garlic, minced

1 cup finely diced white onion

2 cups collard greens, julienned

Sea salt, to taste

3 tablespoons oat flour

½ cup (2 percent) cow's or goat's milk

¾ cup Vegetable Stock*

1 tablespoon ghee

10 cups roughly chopped baby spinach

Roasted Broccoli and Tomatoes

1 head broccoli

2 pints cherry tomatoes

2 teaspoons olive oil

Sea salt, to taste

1 clove garlic

1 tablespoon finely chopped basil

1. Preheat oven to 375 degrees.

2. Dice broccoli into bite-size pieces and toss with tomatoes, olive oil, and sea salt. Place on a sheet pan or in a baking dish and roast for 25 minutes.

3. Remove from oven, and add garlic. Toss to evenly coat, and roast an additional 5 to 10 minutes, until tomatoes are collapsed and blistered and broccoli has slightly crispy, brown edges.

4. Remove from oven and garnish with basil.

▶ SERVES 4

tip: Eating tomatoes and broccoli together in the same dish increases the body's ability to absorb the nutrients that each vegetable supplies.

EAT RIGHT FOR YOUR TYPE PERSONALIZED COOKBOOK

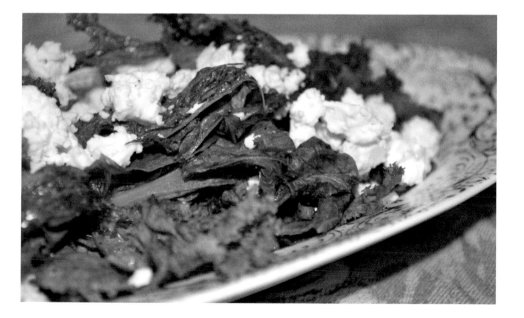
1. Preheat oven to 375 degrees.

2. Wash mustard greens and pat dry with a kitchen towel.

3. Remove greens from woody stems and discard stems. Roughly chop leaves or tear into bite-size pieces. Toss with olive oil, sea salt, and chili powder. Spread on a baking sheet and place on the top rack of the oven.

4. Bake 12 minutes, until greens are wilted with some crispy pieces or edges.

5. Transfer to a serving bowl and add crumbled feta.

6. Serve warm.

1 large bunch mustard greens

2 teaspoons olive oil

½ teaspoon sea salt

1 teaspoon chili powder

½ cup feta cheese, crumbled

▶ SERVES 4

Whipped Sweet Potato Soufflé (NS)

1½ cups (2 percent) cow's or goat's milk

2 sprigs plus 1 tablespoon fresh sage

3 large egg yolks

¼ cup brown rice or spelt flour

1 tablespoon maple syrup (NS substitute agave)

1 cup sweet potato, baked

1 tablespoon ghee plus more for greasing

¼ teaspoon cinnamon

1 teaspoon sea salt

6 egg whites

1. Preheat oven to 350 degrees. Grease bottoms and sides of 8 (4-oz.) ramekins, and set aside.

2. In a small saucepan, gently warm milk with 2 sprigs sage over low heat for 10 to 12 minutes.

3. Whisk egg yolks, brown rice flour, and maple syrup. When milk is ready, temper egg yolks by very slowly pouring about ½ cup warm milk into the egg mixture, stirring continuously. Pour tempered eggs back into the saucepan with the remaining milk, and stir over medium heat until thickened, 2 to 3 minutes.

4. Finely chop remaining 1 tablespoon sage.

5. In a medium bowl, beat baked sweet potato with ghee, fresh sage (finely chopped), cinnamon, and salt. Whisk sweet potato mixture into milk mixture until smooth, and cool completely.

6. In a dry glass, stainless steel, or copper bowl, beat egg whites until they form stiff peaks. Fold egg whites into cooled sweet potato mixture, one-third at a time. Once the egg whites are completely incorporated, spoon batter into prepared ramekins, filling each ramekin three-quarters full.

7. Place ramekins in a large, 2-inch-deep baking dish, and place in the oven with the oven rack extended out of the oven. Pour hot water into the bottom of the baking dish to reach 1 inch. Bake soufflés for 55 to 60 minutes or until firm.

8. Serve immediately.

▶ SERVES 6

Roasted Escarole NS

2 heads escarole,
washed and dried

2 teaspoons olive oil

¼ teaspoon large-grain
sea salt

1. Preheat oven to 375 degrees.

2. Trim woody stems off the bottom of escarole and roughly chop leaves. Toss with olive oil and season with sea salt.

3. Spread escarole on two baking sheets and bake for 10 to 12 minutes. Toss with tongs after 5 minutes, to help the escarole become crispy. Escarole should be dark green, wilted, and have crispy, slightly browned edges.

4. Serve immediately.

▶ SERVES 4

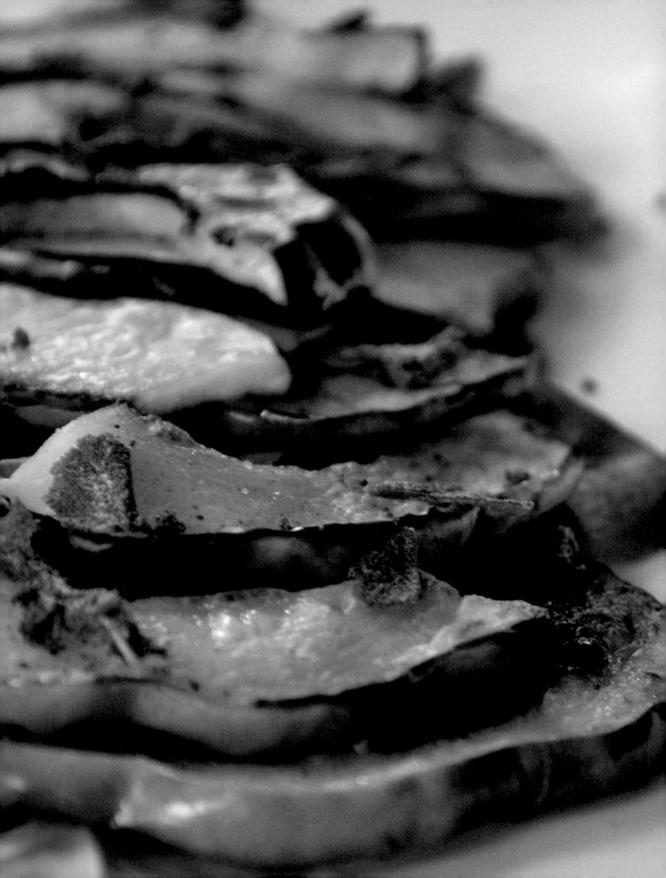

Roasted Pumpkin with Fried Sage NS

1. Preheat oven to 400 degrees.

2. Very carefully cut top off the pumpkin, and slice pumpkin in half vertically. Use a large metal spoon to remove all seeds and membrane from the pumpkin's cavity. Turn pumpkin halves cut side down on a cutting board for stability, and slice into ½-inch sections. Line pumpkin in a single layer on a baking sheet, and drizzle with 2 teaspoons olive oil, a dash of sea salt, and nutmeg.

3. Roast for 45 to 50 minutes or until fork-tender.

4. In the last few minutes of cooking, heat remaining 1 tablespoon olive oil in a small skillet over medium heat. Inspect sage leaves, and dry thoroughly if any water clings to them. (Wetness will splatter the hot oil.) Add sage and fry until crispy, 30 seconds. Remove with a slotted spoon to a paper towel, crumble, and set aside.

5. Remove the pumpkin, garnish with sage, and serve immediately.

▶ SERVES 4

1 (4-lb.) sugar pumpkin

1 tablespoon plus 2 teaspoons olive oil

Sea salt, to taste

⅛ teaspoon nutmeg

2 tablespoons fresh sage

tip: When choosing a pumpkin to roast, opt for a smaller sugar pumpkin, which lends a sweeter flavor. Make sure there are no bruises or weak spots in the flesh and that it feels firm. Additionally, the older the pumpkin is, the firmer and more difficult to cut the skin becomes, so the fresher the better.

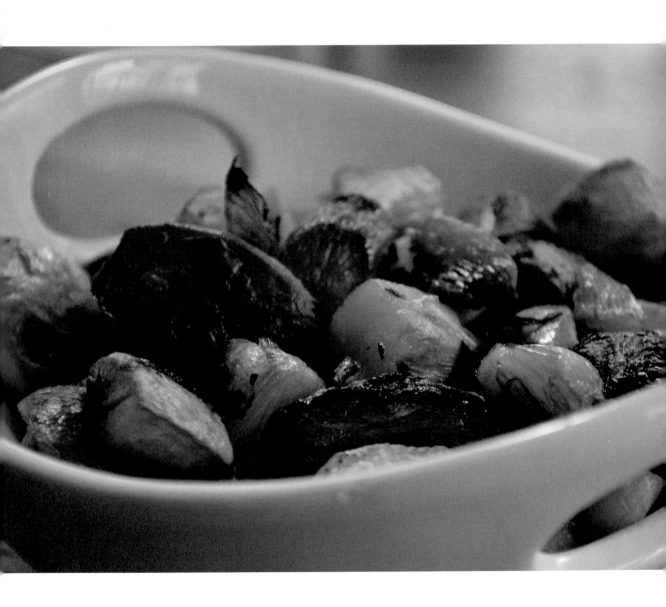

1. Preheat oven to 400 degrees.

2. Peel celery root, turnip, and carrots, and dice into 2-inch pieces.

3. Toss vegetables, cauliflower, shallots, olive oil, sea salt, and sage in a large bowl until evenly coated.

4. Pour onto a baking sheet and bake for 55 to 60 minutes. Vegetables will be browned and crispy on the edges and soft inside.

5. Serve warm.

▶ SERVES 4

1 celery root
1 turnip
2 carrots
2 cups cauliflower florets
4 shallots, diced
1 tablespoon olive oil
1 teaspoon sea salt
2 tablespoons chopped fresh sage

featured ingredient

celery root

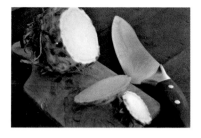

Otherwise known as celeriac, celery root is just what it seems: the root of a type of celery. It has a deliciously fresh flavor that is a cross between celery and parsley, but works terrifically as a base for soups with onions and carrots, eaten raw, or roasted. A *Neutral* for all blood types, celery root adds a diversity of flavor to your palate.

 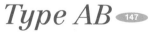

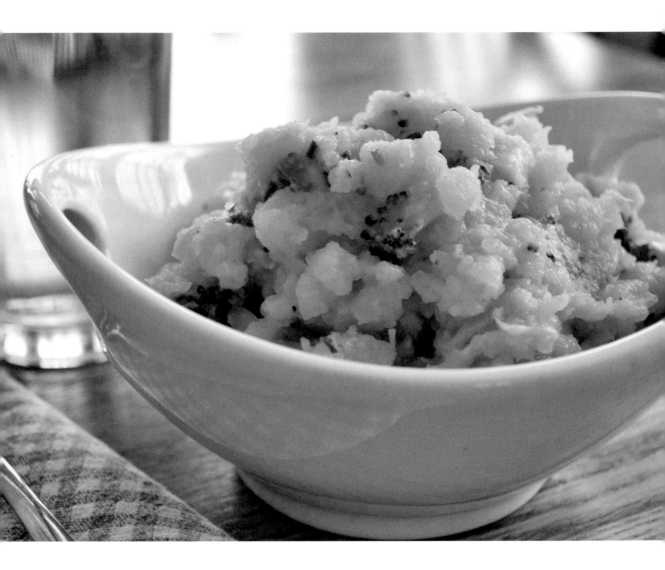

1. Peel rutabagas and dice into 1-inch pieces. Place rutabaga in a pot with enough cold, salted water to cover and bring to a boil. Cover, reduce heat, and simmer for 35 minutes, or until rutabaga is fork-tender.

2. Trim stems off broccoli, and dice into bite-size pieces.

3. Bring another pot of water to boil and steam broccoli for 5 to 6 minutes, until bright green and slightly tender. Drain, and set aside.

4. Drain rutabaga and return it to the pot, placing it back on the burner. Use a potato masher or fork to mash rutabaga, and add parsley, milk, garlic, ghee, and salt. Cook 3 to 4 minutes, until ghee melts and flavors incorporate. Fold broccoli into rutabaga mash.

5. Serve warm.

▶ SERVES 4

2 rutabaga roots
½ teaspoon olive oil
1 head broccoli
¼ cup roughly chopped parsley
¼ cup (2 percent) cow's or goat's milk
2 cloves garlic, peeled
2 teaspoons ghee
Sea salt, to taste

Sweet Potato Hash with Turkey Sausage

6 cups sliced sweet potatoes

2 teaspoons ghee

1 cup diced onion

1 cup diced green bell pepper

2 links turkey sausage

2 teaspoons olive oil

½ teaspoon ground cinnamon

1 tablespoon maple syrup (NS substitute agave)

Sea salt, to taste

1. Slice sweet potatoes into about 2-inch by ¼-inch matchsticks. Place sweet potatoes in a large pot with enough cold water to cover, and bring to a boil. As soon as the water boils, drain and spread sweet potatoes out on a baking sheet lined with a kitchen towel and let dry.

2. Melt ghee in a large skillet over medium heat, and sauté onion and bell pepper for 3 to 4 minutes, until tender.

3. Remove sausages from casing. Add to onion mixture, breaking apart with a flat spatula, and brown, 5-6 minutes. Remove mixture from skillet and set aside.

4. In same skillet, heat olive oil over medium heat. Add sweet potatoes and cook, undisturbed, for 2 minutes to brown potatoes. Flip and cook, undisturbed, for another 2 to 3 minutes to brown the opposite side. Return sausage mixture to skillet, add cinnamon and maple syrup, and stir gently, just to combine. Season with sea salt to taste.

5. Serve hot.

▶ SERVES 6

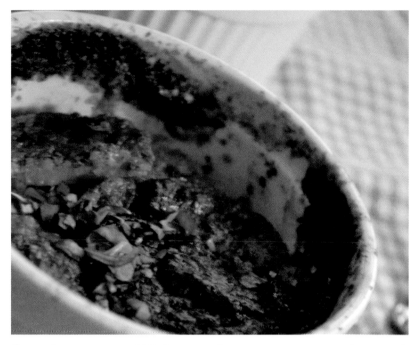

Sweet Potato Gratin with Sage-Walnut Cream NS

2 large sweet potatoes

¾ cup (2 percent) cow's or goat's milk

⅛ teaspoon ground cloves

2 tablespoons fresh sage

½ cup chopped walnuts

Sea salt, to taste

1 cup grated mozzarella or Gruyère cheese

1. Preheat oven to 375 degrees. Spray 2 (12-oz.) ramekins with nonstick cooking spray and set aside.

2. Scrub sweet potatoes and trim off woody ends. Slice into ¼-inch-thick rounds, and place in a bowl of cold water.

3. In a small saucepan, combine milk, cloves, and sage over medium heat, and bring to a simmer.

4. Place walnuts in a food processor and pulse until finely chopped. Gradually drizzle in half of the hot milk mixture and puree until smooth. Add sea salt, to taste.

5. Drain sweet potatoes, and place on a kitchen towel to dry. Spoon a small amount of walnut cream in the bottom of each prepared ramekins. Alternate layers of sweet potato with walnut cream and shredded cheese. Repeat layers until each ramekin is filled to the top, finishing with cream and cheese. Pour remaining milk mixture evenly over each ramekin and bake for 30 to 35 minutes, until potatoes are tender and the cheese is melted and slightly browned.

6. Serve warm.

▶ SERVES 4

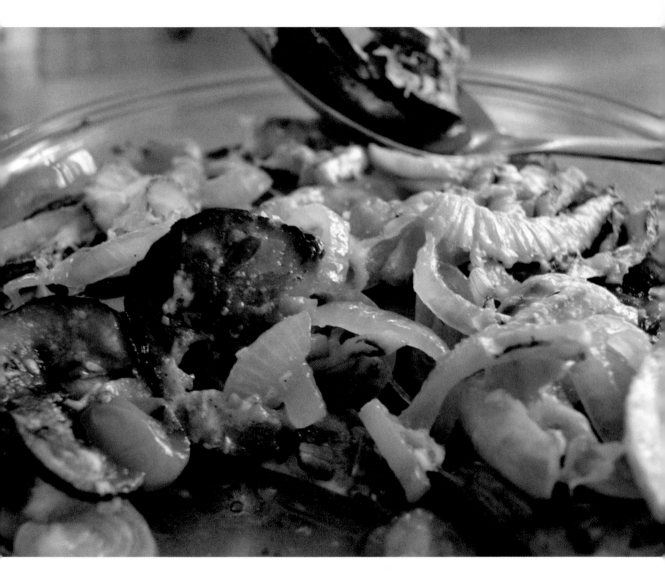

1. Preheat oven to 375 degrees.

2. Slice eggplant into ¼-inch rounds, set on a towel, and sprinkle with sea salt to draw out excess moisture. Slice fennel, tomatoes, and onion into ¼-inch rounds, and set aside.

3. Heat 2 teaspoons olive oil in a large skillet over medium heat. Carefully brown fennel and onion, ensuring vegetables remain in a single layer, 2 to 3 minutes per side. Remove from skillet and set aside.

4. Remove firm base from maitake mushroom and discard. Clean the rest of mushroom with a damp paper towel. Roughly chop into bite-size pieces and sauté in the same skillet set over medium heat for 3 minutes, remove from heat, and set aside.

5. Pat excess moisture off eggplant slices and brown in the same skillet over medium heat, cooking 2 to 3 minutes per side, adding additional oil if necessary. Remove from pan and set aside.

6. Sauté tomatoes, parsley, and garlic in remaining olive oil in pan over medium-high heat for 3 to 4 minutes, allowing some of the liquid from the tomatoes to evaporate.

7. Layer eggplant across the bottom of an 8" × 8" baking dish, and top with tomato mixture and ¼ cup cheese. Top with onion, fennel, maitake, and remaining ¼ cup cheese.

8. Bake, uncovered, for 20 minutes. Vegetables will be soft and cheese will be melted. Serve warm or let come to room temperature, store in refrigerator, and serve cold.

▶ SERVES 4

1 medium eggplant

Sea salt, to taste

1 bulb fennel

2 cups mini heirloom tomatoes

1 large white onion

1 tablespoon olive oil, divided

1 maitake mushroom

½ cup chopped parsley

2 cloves garlic

½ cup hard goat cheese, grated

Tomato-Broccoli Ragu NS

2 teaspoons olive oil

1 cup finely diced onion

1 cup finely diced carrots

1 cup finely diced celery

½ cup finely diced parsnips

1 clove garlic, minced

I cup broccoli florets

3 vine-ripened tomatoes, diced

½ cup Vegetable Stock*

Sea salt, to taste

1 cup Rice Polenta*

¼ cup chopped basil for garnish

1. Heat olive oil in a large sauté pan over medium heat. Add onion, carrots, celery, and parsnips, and sauté 5 to 6 minutes, until vegetables begin to soften.

2. Add garlic, broccoli, tomatoes, and stock, and season with sea salt, to taste. Bring to a boil, reduce heat, and simmer for 30 minutes, stirring occasionally, until vegetables are fork-tender.

3. Serve warm, on top of creamy Rice Polenta, and garnish with basil.

*See Vegetable Stock NS recipe (page 221). See Rice Polenta NS recipe (page 155).

▶ SERVES 4

1. Cook farina according to package instructions. Two minutes before farina is finished cooking, add remaining ingredients, stirring constantly.

2. Serve immediately.

▶ SERVES 2

½ cup brown rice farina

1 teaspoon dried parsley

¼ cup mozzarella cheese

2 teaspoons olive oil

½ teaspoon onion powder

tip: If farina is ready before the rest of your meal and becomes too thick, simply add warm water, 1 tablespoon at a time, until desired consistency is achieved.

Brown Rice Salad NS

¾ cup brown rice

1½ cups water

2 teaspoons olive oil

½ cup diced celery

1 tablespoon fresh sage

1 cup diced maitake mushrooms

1 cup diced silver dollar mushrooms

¼ cup finely diced shallots

2 cups arugula

2 tablespoons toasted almonds

1. Cook brown rice in water according to package instructions. Set aside and let cool slightly.

2. Heat olive oil in a medium skillet over medium heat and sauté celery, sage, mushrooms, and shallots for 3 to 4 minutes, until vegetables begin to soften.

3. In a large serving bowl, toss brown rice, mushroom mixture, arugula, and toasted almonds. The brown rice will be warm and will wilt the arugula slightly.

4. Serve warm or at room temperature.

▶ SERVES 4

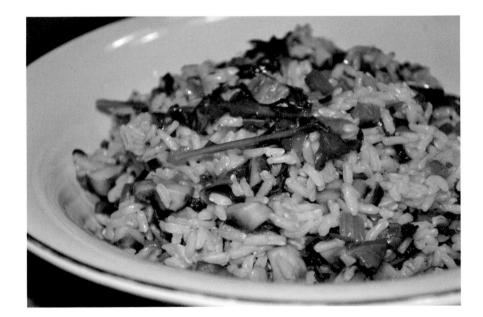

1. Heat olive oil in a Dutch oven over medium heat, and sauté onion and rice for 3 to 4 minutes, stirring constantly.

2. In a small pot, heat stock and milk. Slowly add one ladle of liquid at a time to the rice and onions, until liquid is almost absorbed. Add the next ladle, and repeat until all the liquid has been used, about 1 hour . Season with sea salt, to taste.

3. Serve warm.

*See Vegetable Stock NS recipe (page 221).

▶ SERVES 4

2 teaspoons olive oil

½ cup finely diced white onion

1 cup forbidden black rice

2 cups Vegetable Stock*

¾ cup (2 percent) cow's or goat's milk

½ teaspoon sea salt

 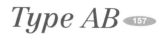

Herbed Quinoa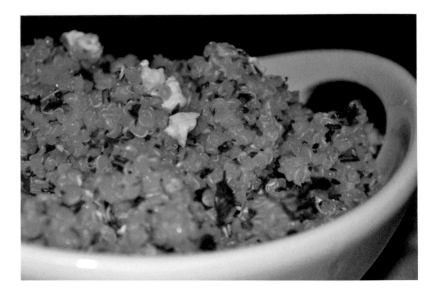

1 cup quinoa

1 cup Vegetable Stock*

1 cup water

1 tablespoon fresh rosemary, chopped

1 tablespoon fresh thyme, chopped

1 tablespoon fresh parsley, chopped

½ teaspoon lemon zest

2 tablespoons flaxseed

¼ cup crumbled feta cheese

1. Combine quinoa, stock, and water in a pot, bring to a boil, reduce heat, and simmer for 10 to 12 minutes, until water is absorbed and quinoa is soft and tender.

2. Fluff cooked quinoa with a fork and toss with rosemary, thyme, parsley, lemon zest, flaxseed, and feta cheese. Serve warm.

*See Vegetable Stock NS recipe (page 221).

▶ SERVES 4

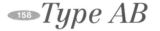
EAT RIGHT FOR YOUR TYPE PERSONALIZED COOKBOOK

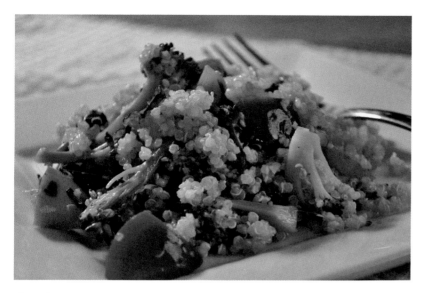

Crisp-Tender Veggie Quinoa NS

1 small head broccoli

1 bunch rappini

1 (4-inch) piece lemongrass

1 cup quinoa

2 cups water

Sea salt, to taste

2 teaspoons olive oil

1 cup cherry tomatoes, halved

2 teaspoons lemon zest

1. Chop broccoli and rappini into bite-size pieces. Bring a large pot of water to a boil and cook broccoli and rappini, 3 minutes. Remove vegetables with a slotted spoon and place in an ice bath to stop the cooking process. Drain and set aside on a kitchen towel.

2. Bruise lemongrass by hammering with the back of your knife, just until aromatic. Bring quinoa and water to a boil with a pinch of salt, and reduce heat to simmer. Add lemongrass to the quinoa, and cook 12 minutes.

3. Heat olive oil in a large skillet over medium heat, and sauté broccoli and rappini, 3 to 4 minutes, until vegetables are crisp-tender and bright green. Remove lemongrass from cooked quinoa, and toss broccoli, rappini, tomatoes, and lemon zest with quinoa. Add sea salt, to taste.

4. Serve warm or cold.

▶ SERVES 6

 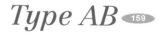

Mint and Cherry Tomato Tabbouleh

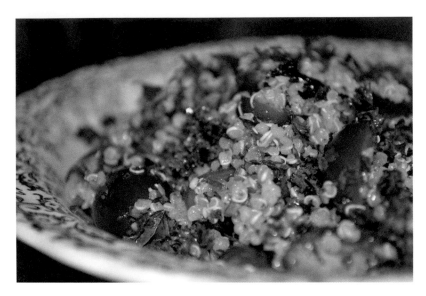

1 cup quinoa

2 cups water

Sea salt, to taste

3 tablespoons olive oil, divided

4 cups torn kale

1 tablespoon lemon juice

1 tablespoon lemon zest

2 cloves garlic, minced

¾ cup mint

2 cups parsley

1½ cups halved cherry tomatoes

1. Preheat oven to 400 degrees.

2. In a saucepan, combine quinoa, water, and add a dash of sea salt. Bring to a boil, cover, reduce heat, and simmer for 10 minutes. Remove from heat and leave covered an additional 4 to 5 minutes, until all the water is absorbed and quinoa is tender and fluffy. Fluff with a fork and set aside to cool.

3. While the quinoa cooks, drizzle 2 teaspoons olive oil over kale on a baking sheet and sprinkle with sea salt. Bake for 10 to 12 minutes, until kale pieces are crispy.

4. Whisk remaining olive oil, lemon juice, lemon zest, and garlic in a large bowl. Add mint, parsley, tomatoes, quinoa, and kale, and toss to evenly distribute dressing.

5. Serve room temperature or chilled.

▶ SERVES 6

Snacks

Snacks are the most difficult place for most people to get creative and come up with new ideas that are not overly complicated. We hope you find in this chapter a few new options that will make snacking easier, tastier, and healthier. There are also a few snacks that translate well as appetizers if you like entertaining or have a little extra time to prepare something special.

Toasty Pizza Bites NS

2 teaspoons olive oil

½ cup finely chopped white onion

4 vine-ripened tomatoes, seeded and chopped

1 clove garlic, minced

1 teaspoon agave

Sea salt, to taste

1 tablespoon chopped fresh basil

2 slices spelt or oat bread

2 thin slices fresh mozzarella cheese

½ teaspoon dried oregano

1. Heat olive oil in a skillet set over medium and sauté onion, 5 to 6 minutes. Add tomatoes, garlic, and agave, and season with sea salt. Simmer for 8 to 10 minutes, until tomatoes and onion become soft and melt into a slightly thickened sauce. Stir in basil and remove from heat.

2. Lightly toast bread and spread tomato sauce on toast, top with mozzarella cheese, and garnish with oregano. Place pizza under the broiler for 1 to 2 minutes or until cheese is melted and bubbling. Keep an eye on the pizza so the cheese does not burn.

3. Serve warm.

▶ SERVES 2

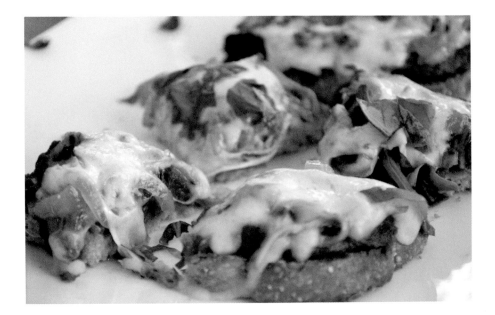

Heirloom Tomato and Eggplant Salsa

1. Bring a large pot of water to a gentle boil. Using a paring knife, make a X on the top of each tomato, place tomatoes into pot, and submerge for up to 1 minute. Remove with a slotted spoon and let cool. The skin of the tomato should peel away easily. Chop tomatoes and set aside.

2. Heat olive oil in a large skillet over medium heat. Add eggplant and sauté eggplant for 5 to 6 minutes. Add garlic and onion and sauté an additional 5 minutes. Add tomatoes and cilantro, stir to combine, and cook for 5 minutes. Season with sea salt, to taste.

3. Serve warm or let cool completely, refrigerate, and serve chilled.

▶ SERVES 4

tip: Parsley can be substituted for cilantro in equal amounts in this recipe.

4 large heirloom tomatoes

2 teaspoons olive oil

1 cup chopped eggplant

1 clove garlic, minced

1 cup diced white onion

¼ cup cilantro

½ teaspoon sea salt

Crudités and Creamy Goat Cheese Dip NS

dip:

4 ounces soft goat cheese

2 tablespoons chopped dill

2 teaspoons agave

½ teaspoon sea salt

1 tablespoon lemon juice

1 tablespoon (2 percent) cow's or goat's milk

crudités:

Baby carrots

Celery sticks

Kohlrabi sticks

1. Whisk all dip ingredients in a bowl until smooth and fully incorporated. Spoon into a serving dish, and plate with vegetables.

▶ SERVES 4

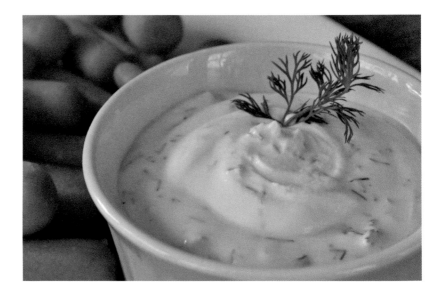

1. Place all ingredients in a food processor or mini-chopper and puree until smooth and creamy.

2. Serve immediately or chill in the refrigerator until ready to eat. Serve with Flax Crackers NS (page 167) or crudités.

▶ SERVES 4

1½ cups cooked (or canned) navy beans, drained and rinsed

½ cup chopped fresh basil

2 tablespoons chopped fresh parsley

1 clove garlic, minced

2 teaspoons olive oil

1 tablespoon walnuts

1 teaspoon lemon zest

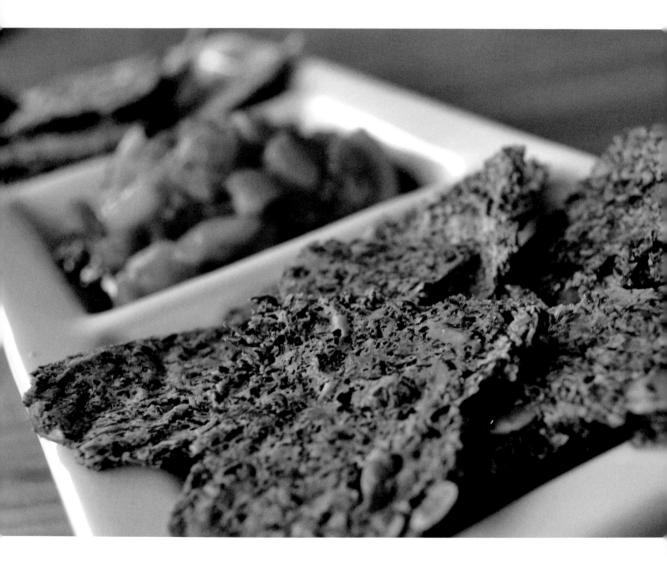

1. Combine flaxseed with water, stir, and set aside for 15 minutes. Mixture will become thick and goopy.

2. Preheat oven to 200 degrees. Line a 15" × 10" baking sheet with parchment paper and set aside.

3. Add sea salt and walnuts to soaked flaxseed, stirring to combine. Mixture will be slightly thicker in consistency than cake batter. Pour flax mixture onto the center of the sheet. Spray an offset spatula with cooking spray or coat with olive oil to help you spread the flax mixture without sticking. Spread flax mixture in a thin layer as evenly as possible across entire baking sheet.

4. Bake for 2 hours. Crackers will solidify and be slightly rubbery in texture.

5. Increase the oven temperature to 400 degrees and bake 10 minutes to make the crackers crispy. Carefully flip the crackers and bake an additional 5 to 6 minutes. When done, crackers will be hardened and crispy on both sides. Let cool and break apart into pieces the size of tortilla chips. Serve room temperature and store in a cool, dry place or in the freezer.

▶ SERVES 4

1 cup ground flaxseed
⅔ cup hot water
¼ teaspoon sea salt
¼ cup finely ground walnuts

tip: Whole flaxseed will last longer than ground, so buy whole and grind in a coffee grinder or food processor when needed to maximize shelf life.

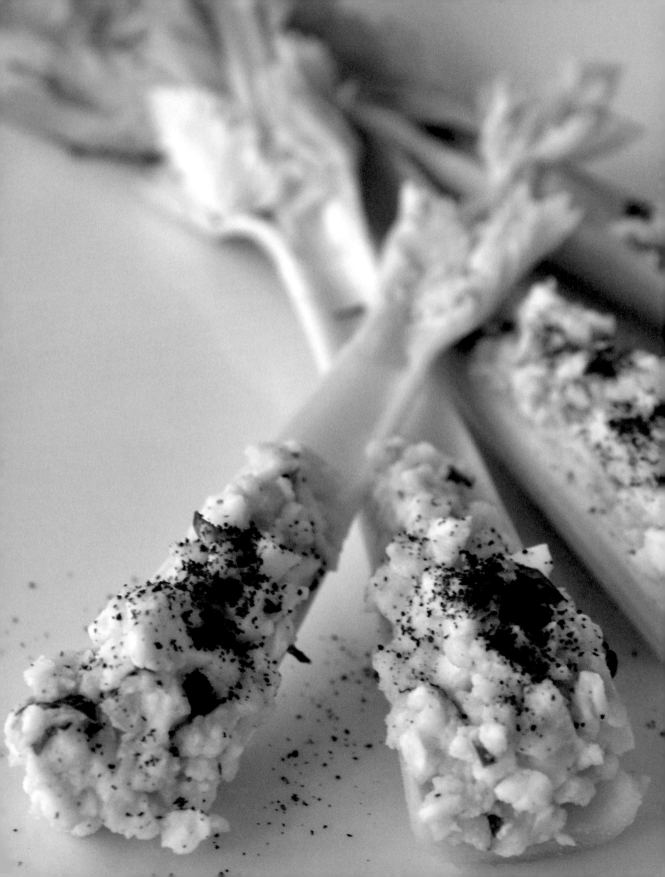

1. Place eggs in a saucepan and cover with cold water. Bring to a boil and turn off the heat. Set a timer for 14 minutes and when done, rinse eggs under cold water. Peel eggs, chop, and place them in a large bowl.

2. Add remaining ingredients to eggs and toss to combine.

3. Serve egg salad on celery sticks or between slices of brown rice toast.

▶ SERVES 4

4 large eggs

½ teaspoon dried mustard

1 tablespoon chopped parsley

¼ teaspoon sea salt

½ teaspoon curry powder

⅛ teaspoon turmeric

2 teaspoons olive oil

2 teaspoons lemon juice

Farmer Cheese and Beet-Endive Cups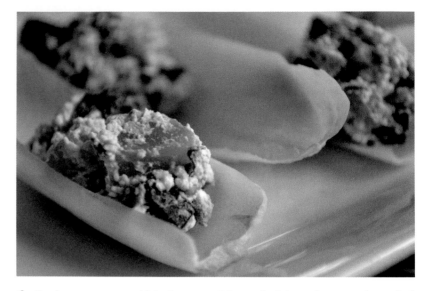

2 medium orange beets
2 medium red beets
2 teaspoons olive oil
¼ cup farmer cheese
¼ cup chopped walnuts
1 teaspoon lemon juice
Sea salt, to taste
2 heads endive

1. Preheat oven to 400 degrees. Line a baking sheet with tinfoil and set aside.

2. Trim tops and bottoms off beets and scrub clean. Place on prepared baking sheet, coat with olive oil and bake for 60 to 65 minutes or until easily pierced with a knife.

3. Let beets cool for 10 minutes. Carefully remove skin with a paring knife, and dice into ½-inch cubes. Place in a bowl and add farmer cheese, walnuts, and lemon juice. Season to taste with sea salt, and toss to combine.

4. Spoon about 2 teaspoons filling onto each endive leaf.

5. Serve immediately or chill, covered, in the refrigerator until ready to serve.

▶ SERVES 4

tip: Store-bought, precooked beets, either canned or in vacuum-sealed packages in the produce department can be substituted in this recipe, but beets from a can may be exposed to BPA's and tend to lose a great deal of flavor and sweetness.

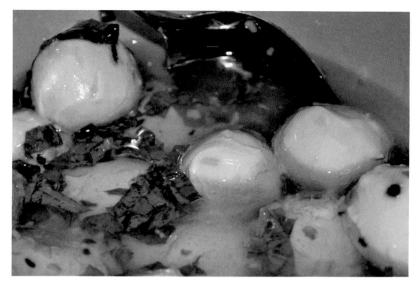

Marinated Mozzarella

NS

½ cup extra virgin olive oil

1 teaspoon large-grain sea salt

2 cloves garlic, minced

2 tablespoons chopped basil

2 kalamata olives, pitted and finely diced

1 pound fresh mozzarella balls

1. Place olive oil, sea salt, garlic, basil, and olives in a medium-size bowl and stir well. Add mozzarella balls, toss to coat, and refrigerate for 2 hours or more.

2. Remove from refrigerator 15 minutes before serving, to allow oil to come to room temperature.

3. Marinated mozzarella will keep in refrigerator for up to 1 week.

▶ SERVES 4

tip: If you cannot find individually portioned miniature mozzarella balls, buy 1 large ball of fresh cheese and cut into 1–2-inch pieces as a substitute.

Spicy Rosemary-Nut Clusters

2 tablespoons fresh rosemary

1 teaspoon chili powder

½ teaspoon salt

1 tablespoon maple syrup (NS substitute agave)

2 teaspoons ghee

1 cup quartered black or English walnuts

½ cup roughly chopped pecans

½ cup crushed almonds

1. Preheat oven to 325 degrees.

2. Toss all ingredients in a bowl and spread on a baking sheet. Bake for 25 minutes, tossing once halfway through. Nuts will be aromatic and lightly browned when done. Let cool and spoon into a bowl to serve.

3. Store in a cool, dry place for up to 1 week.

▶ SERVES 6

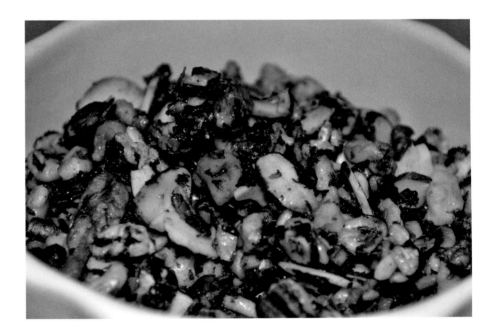

EAT RIGHT FOR YOUR TYPE PERSONALIZED COOKBOOK

1. Preheat oven to 400 degrees.

2. Spread cauliflower and garlic in a single layer on a sheet pan. Drizzle with olive oil and sea salt (do not salt too heavily, as feta cheese is salty). Roast for 30 minutes, until cauliflower is fork-tender. Remove garlic and set aside.

3. Toss cauliflower with spinach in a bowl to wilt spinach slightly. Rub roasted garlic evenly on 3 pieces of toast and slice toast in quarters.

4. Add feta cheese to cauliflower and spinach and spoon evenly over toast to serve.

▶ SERVES 2

1½ cups cauliflower florets

2 cloves garlic

1 tablespoon olive oil, divided

Sea salt, to taste

2 cups chopped spinach

3 slices brown rice or spelt bread

¼ cup feta cheese, crumbled

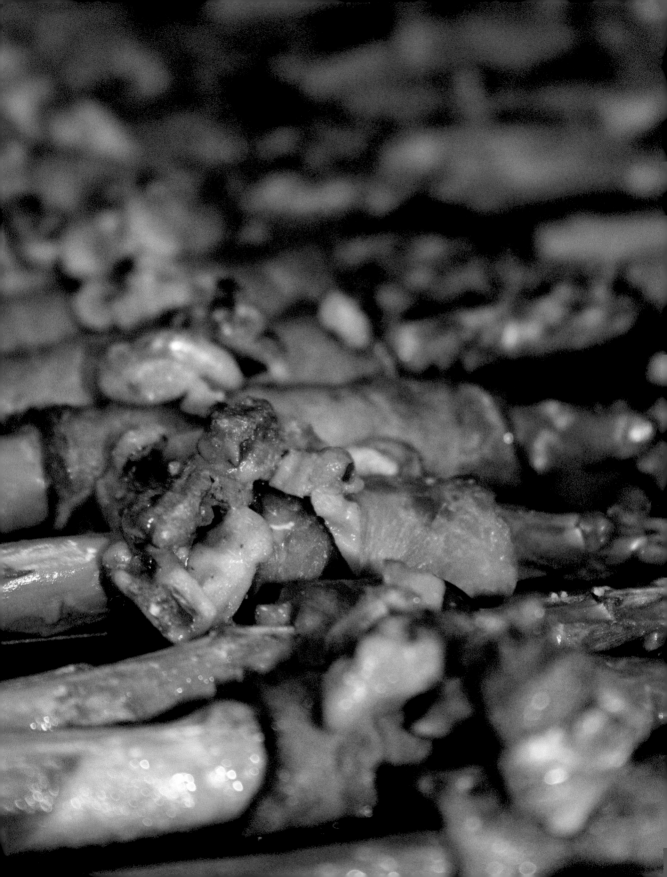

Asparagus Wrapped with Crispy Walnut Bacon

1. Preheat oven to 375 degrees. Grease a wire rack with nonstick cooking spray and set aside.

2. In a small bowl, combine maple syrup, ground ginger, and walnuts, and set aside.

3. Prepare asparagus by cutting off and discarding woody bottoms. Toss with olive oil. Slice bacon lengthwise and then into thirds. Wrap bacon around each spear of asparagus and place on prepared wire rack. Repeat until all asparagus is wrapped.

4. Place wire rack lined with asparagus on a baking sheet. Spoon the maple-walnut mixture over asparagus.

5. Bake for 10 to 12 minutes on middle rack, until walnuts begin to smell nutty and edges of bacon are crispy. Serve warm.

▶ SERVES 4

2 tablespoons maple syrup (NS substitute agave)

1 teaspoon ground ginger

½ cup chopped walnuts

1 bunch asparagus spears

5 slices nitrate-/preservative-free turkey bacon

2 teaspoons olive oil

Crispy Spring Vegetable Cakes NS

1 small celery root, peeled

1 small bulb fennel

2 tablespoons grated onion

2 cups spinach

½ teaspoon lemon zest

1 tablespoon chopped sage

1 large egg, beaten

2 tablespoons spelt flour

⅓ cup bread crumbs*

2 teaspoons olive oil

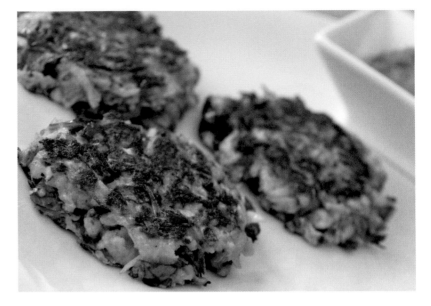

1. Use a food processor or a hand grater to shred celery root and fennel. Place celery root, fennel, and onion in a bowl. Finely chop spinach and add to vegetables with lemon zest, sage, egg, flour, and bread crumbs. Toss to combine.

2. Heat olive oil in a large skillet set over medium heat. Using an ice cream scoop, spoon vegetable mixture into pan, allowing 1 inch between each vegetable cake. Cook 2 to 3 minutes, flip, and cook an additional 2 to 3 minutes. Cakes should be brown and crispy on each side and warm and tender in the center, but cooked through.

3. Serve warm.

*See Basic Bread Crumbs recipe (page 222).

▶ SERVES 4

tip: As an alternative serving option, cool and refrigerate vegetable cakes, and eat for breakfast topped with a poached or fried egg.

1. Peel apples and dice into 1-inch cubes.

2. Combine apples, cinnamon stick, apple juice, and cranberries in a saucepan set over medium heat. Add 1 tablespoon agave; add up to 1 additional tablespoon depending on the tartness of the apples and cranberries. Cook for 30 minutes, or until apples no longer hold their shape, stirring occasionally.

3. Remove from heat, and serve warm or chilled.

▶ SERVES 6

2 organic Red Delicious apples (about 2 cups diced)

2 organic Granny Smith apples (about 2 cups diced)

1 cinnamon stick

½ cup apple juice

½ cup frozen or fresh organic cranberries

1–2 tablespoons agave

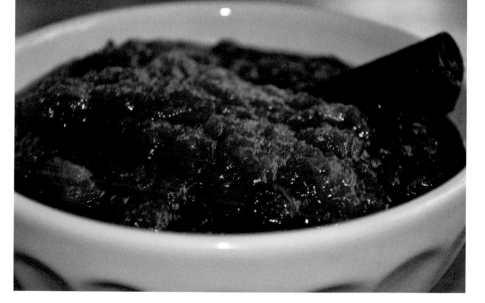

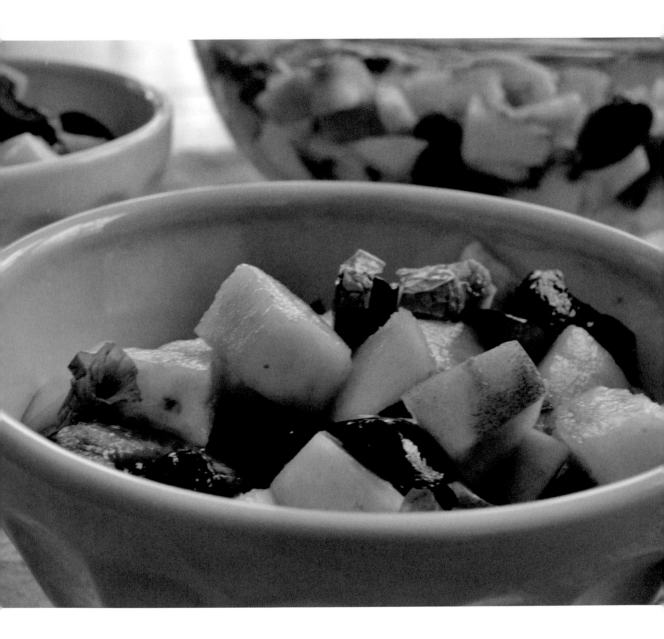

Fruit Salad with Mint-Lime Dressing (NS)

1. Place dried cranberries in a small bowl. Cover with hot water and steep for 10 minutes, to rehydrate.

2. Peel and dice peaches, pineapple, and kiwi into ½-inch pieces and toss with cherries in a large serving bowl.

3. Strain cranberries from water and gently pat dry on a kitchen towel. Add to fruit salad.

4. Whisk lime zest and juice, agave, and mint leaves in a small bowl. Pour over fruit salad toss, and serve chilled.

▶ SERVES 4

½ cup dried cranberries

2 organic peaches

1 pineapple

4 kiwis

2 cups fresh cherries, quartered

Zest and juice of 2 limes

1 teaspoon agave

½ cup finely chopped mint leaves

Pear and Apple Chips

2 Bosc pears

2 Bartlett pears

2 Braeburn apples

¼ teaspoon cinnamon

1. Preheat oven to 225 degrees. Line a baking sheet with parchment paper and set aside.

2. Slice pears and apples in rounds as thinly as you can, or use a mandolin to help you. Line sliced fruit in a single layer on the baking sheet, and sprinkle evenly with cinnamon. Bake for 2 hours, flipping fruit halfway through cooking.

3. Cool completely and serve.

▶ SERVES 4

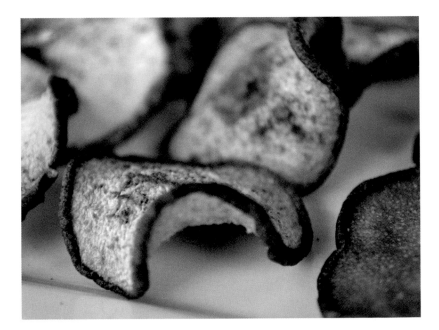

2 whole ruby red grapefruits, halved

2 teaspoons honey

½ teaspoon cinnamon

1. Preheat oven to 400 degrees.

2. Trim the rounded bottom slightly of each grapefruit half, to create a stable base. Place on a baking sheet, cut-flesh side up.

3. Drizzle each half evenly with honey and cinnamon.

4. Bake for 5 to 6 minutes and then broil for 1 to 2 additional minutes, until the edges of the grapefruit are browned and the fruit is hot and topping is bubbling.

▶ SERVES 4

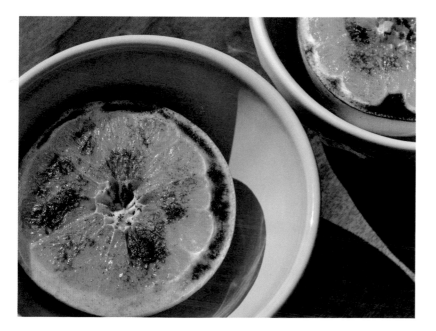

Grilled Pineapple with Cinnamon Syrup

2 teaspoons light olive oil
1 fresh pineapple
¼ cup Cinnamon Syrup*

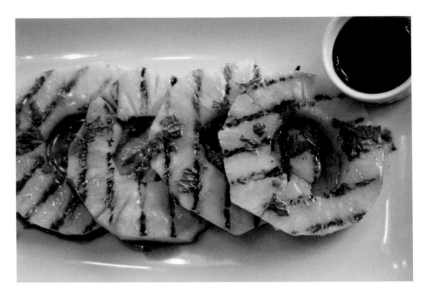

1. Preheat grill pan over medium heat, and brush with oil to create a nonstick surface.

2. Remove outer layer of pineapple, core, and slice into rounds. Brush one side of pineapple rounds with Cinnamon Syrup and place, sauce side down, on the grill pan. Let cook 2 to 3 minutes and brush the opposite side with Cinnamon Syrup.

3. Flip and grill an additional 2 to 3 minutes. Serve warm.

*See Cinnamon Syrup recipe (page 219).

▶ SERVES 4

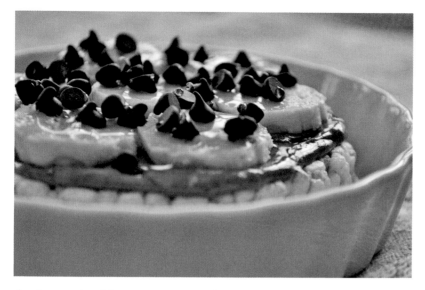

4 tablespoons peanut butter

2 rice cakes

1 small apple, thinly sliced

2 tablespoons mini dark chocolate chips

1 teaspoon honey

1. Smear 2 tablespoons peanut butter on each rice cake and top each with 2 slices of apple, 1 tablespoon chocolate chips, and a drizzle of honey (about ½ teaspoon each).

▶ SERVES 2

Carob–Walnut Butter–Stuffed Figs (NS)

5 fresh or dried figs

¼ cup walnut halves

2 tablespoons pecans

1 tablespoon Carob Extract™* plus more for garnishing

1 teaspoon olive oil

3 tablespoons hot water

Sea salt, to taste

1. Slice figs in half from stem to base.

2. In a food processor, combine walnuts, pecans, Carob Extract™ and olive oil, and puree. As the processor is running, drizzle in hot water so that the mixture forms a thick paste similar in consistency to natural peanut butter. Season with sea salt, to taste.

3. Spoon about 1 teaspoon of the nut butter mixture over each fig half and drizzle with extra Carob Extract™, if desired.

*Information about purchasing Carob Extract™ can be found in Appendix II: Products (page 247).

▶ SERVES 2

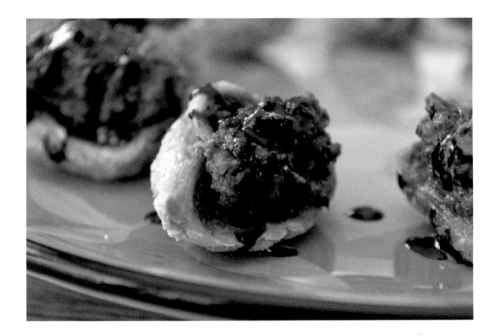

Drinks and Beverages

Any time you start a new diet plan, it is nice to have as many taste and flavor options available to you, especially when you are just getting started. This will help to add diversity to your day in a simple and tasty way. Plus, there are plenty of us who have a routine of drinking coffee or black tea or soda, and these beverage suggestions can help to substitute for the old habits you are trying to kick. Also included in this chapter are recipes for smoothies, which can spice up your snack or breakfast routine, or maybe even replace that milkshake that becomes tempting in the hot, summer months.

Pineapple Spa Water (NS)

2 sprigs mint
6 cup water
4 (¼-inch-thick) pineapple rounds

1. Wash mint and place in a large pitcher with water and pineapple slices. Let chill in refrigerator for 2 to 3 hours.

2. Serve chilled.

▶ SERVES 4

Cherry Spritzer

6 pitted cherries
½ cup mint leaves
½ cup black cherry juice
1 pint seltzer water

1. In a large pitcher, crush cherries and mint leaves. Add cherry juice and seltzer. Serve over ice.

▶ SERVES 4

Type AB

1. Wash and dry vegetables. Cut off tough ends of kale and carrots, and push kale, lemon, carrots, apples, and ginger through juicer, one at a time. Stir together and enjoy.

▶ SERVES 4

tip: Vegetable juices will keep in the refrigerator for up to 3 days, but provide the best nutritional value when consumed immediately after juicing.

1 bunch kale
4 large carrots, peeled
½ lemon
4 apples
1 (3-inch) piece ginger

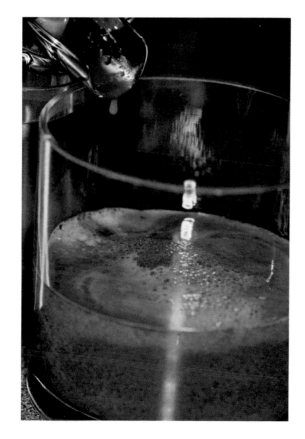

Cooling Chamomile Spritzer NS

4 cups water
½ cup sliced peaches
1 cup mint leaves
4 chamomile tea bags
2 cups sparkling water
¼ cup peach nectar

1. Bring water to a gentle boil and remove from heat.

2. Add peaches, mint leaves, and tea bags, steep for 4 to 5 minutes. Remove tea bags and let cool in refrigerator until chilled, about 1 hour.

3. Add sparkling water and peach nectar, stir, and serve over ice.

▶ SERVES 4

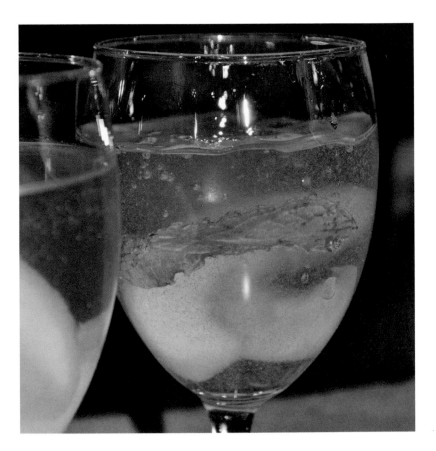

EAT RIGHT FOR YOUR TYPE PERSONALIZED COOKBOOK

1. Heat water almost to a boil. Add mint and lime juice and zest, cover, and steep, 5 minutes.

2. Spoon matcha powder into a heat-safe glass pitcher and gradually add minty water, whisking continuously. Strain the mint and zest out of the tea. Add honey and serve.

▶ SERVES 4

6 cups water

1 cup fresh mint

Zest and juice of 1 lime

2 teaspoons matcha powder

1 tablespoon honey (NS substitute agave)

featured ingredient

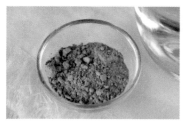

matcha

Matcha is a powdered form of green tea. Once tea leaves are sun dried, they are finely ground and then whisked into not-yet-boiling water. Matcha was originally used as a ceremonial tea in Japan, and has recently become a popular trend in the United States. Because drinking matcha means ingesting all of the tea leaf instead of what is steeped from the leaves, you are consuming a greatly increased amount of antioxidants. Matcha can also be used in baked goods such as cookies and cakes.

Sweet Basil and Ginger Tea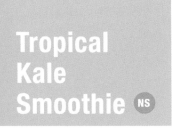

4 cups water

1 (2-inch) piece ginger, peeled and roughly chopped

¼ cup torn basil leaves

1 teaspoon agave nectar

1. Bring water to a boil with ginger, remove from heat, and add basil leaves. Let steep at least 3 minutes. Stir in agave, strain ginger and basil leaves and serve tea warm.

▶ SERVES 2

Tropical Kale Smoothie

1 cup diced frozen pineapple

⅓ cup diced frozen peaches

½ cup frozen blueberries

¼ cup frozen kale

¾ cup grapefruit juice

2 teaspoons agave

2 tablespoons Protein Blend Powder™—Type B/AB*

½ teaspoon ground cinnamon

1. Place all ingredients in a blender and blend until smooth. If you have an immersion blender, place all ingredients in a large blender cup and blend with immersion blender.

*Information about purchasing Protein Blend™ Powder—Type B/AB can be found in Appendix II: Products (page 247).

▶ SERVES 4

EAT RIGHT FOR YOUR TYPE PERSONALIZED COOKBOOK

1. Combine all ingredients in a blender and blend until smooth, pour into 2 glasses, and serve cold.

*Information about purchasing Protein Blend™ Powder—Type B/AB can be found in Appendix II: Products (page 247).

▶ SERVES 2

½ cup raspberries

½ cup pineapple

¾ cup blueberries

1 cup torn kale

1 cup (2 percent) cow's or goat's milk

2 tablespoons peanut butter

2 teaspoons agave

1 tablespoon flaxseed

2 scoops Protein Blend Powder™—Type B/AB*

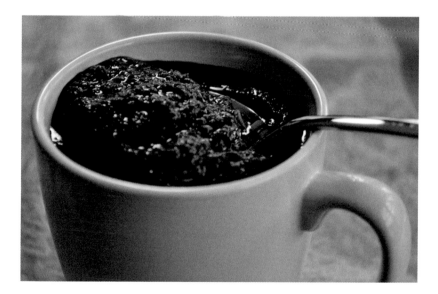

Creamy Almond Butter Smoothie

4 figs

2 tablespoons Protein Blend Powder™—Type B/AB*

1 cup (2 percent) cow's or goat's milk

¼ cup diced frozen pears

1 tablespoon flaxseed

1½ tablespoons almond butter

1. Combine all ingredients in a blender and blend until smooth, or use an immersion blender. For easier blending, add liquid to the blender first. Serve chilled.

*Information about purchasing Protein Blend™ Powder—Type B/AB can be found in Appendix II: Products (page 247).

▶ SERVES 2

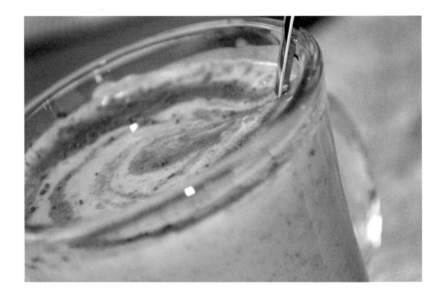

Desserts

Deep-Chocolate Brownies NS ■ *Cherry-Chocolate Fondue* NS ■ *Chocolate Salted-Nut Clusters* NS ■ *Cocoa-Dusted Chocolate Truffles* NS ■ *Fig Bars* NS ■ *Almond-Cranberry Biscotti* NS ■ *Chocolate Chip Cookies* NS ■ *Blueberry Crumble* NS ■ *Peach, Acai, and Cinnamon Charlotte* NS ■ *Carrot-Pineapple Cake with Chocolate Frosting* NS ■ *Upside-Down Almond Cake with Apricot Glaze* ■ *Matcha Cake with Chocolate Frosting* ■ *Creamy Berry Ricotta* NS ■ *Ginger Rice Pudding* ■ *Millet Crêpes with Raspberry Chutney and Chocolate Syrup* NS

What is a cookbook without desserts? The best way to stick to any kind of diet—even ones not meant for weight loss—is to have realistic options for indulging your sweet tooth once in a while. Although these recipes sound indulgent, they are written to be as healthful as possible while still feeling like a satisfying dessert. Whenever possible, use agave or molasses as sweeteners, include allowable grains, limit fats, and feel free to use chocolate.

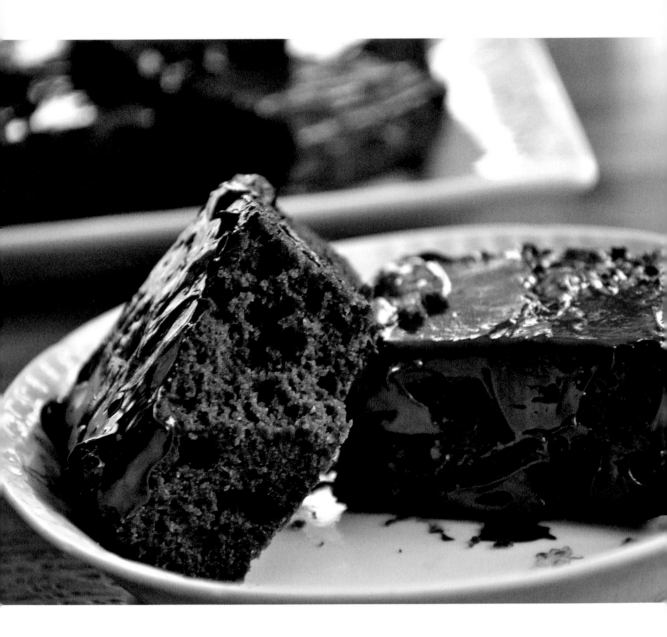

1. Preheat oven to 350 degrees. Grease an 8" × 8" baking dish and set aside.

2. In a large bowl, combine flours, baking powder, sea salt, and cocoa powder. Set aside.

3. In a separate bowl, whisk eggs, applesauce, ghee, and agave. Add the egg mixture to the dry ingredients and stir to combine.

4. If you do not have a double boiler, set a glass bowl on top of a small saucepan filled one-third of the way with water (water should not be touching the bowl). Bring the water to a boil and add shaved chocolate. Let melt and remove from heat. Add chocolate and warm water to batter, stirring to combine.

5. Pour batter into prepared baking pan and bake for 30 to 35 minutes, or until firm to the touch and a cake tester inserted into brownies comes out clean.

6. Remove from oven and turn off the heat. Pour chocolate chips over the top of the brownies and place back into the oven for 2 to 3 minutes. Use an offset spatula to spread melted chips evenly across the top of the brownies. Let cool for 10 minutes, slice, and serve warm.

7. Brownies will stay in a cool, dry place up to 2 days or in the freezer for up to 1 month.

▶ SERVES 8

Deep-Chocolate Brownies NS

1 cup spelt flour

½ cup oat flour

1 teaspoon baking powder

½ teaspoon sea salt

2 tablespoons cocoa powder

2 eggs

¼ cup applesauce

3 tablespoons ghee, melted and cooled, or light olive oil

½ cup agave

2 ounces 100 percent dark chocolate, shaved

¼ cup warm water

½ cup chocolate chips

featured ingredient

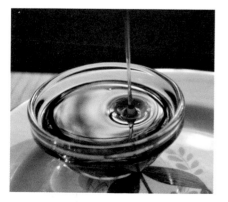

agave nectar

Agave is a natural sweetener derived from the agave plant, commonly found in the southwestern areas of America and in Mexico. Agave is most commonly known for its role as the base ingredient of tequila. It can be used in baking and cooking in place of sugar, however, the agave-to-sugar ratio is not 1:1 because it is a liquid. Agave has a mild taste akin to that of honey, but its flavor is much less noticeable.

Cherry-Chocolate Fondue NS

fondue:

2 ounces 100 percent chocolate, shaved

2 tablespoons agave

1 cup cherry juice

1 tablespoon cherry jam

2 teaspoons ghee

1 cup diced pineapple

1 cup dried apricot

1 cup sliced apples

1. Place chocolate into a mixing bowl, and set aside.

2. In a saucepan, bring agave, juice, jam, and ghee to a simmer and remove from heat. Pour mixture over chocolate and stir to combine.

3. Serve with fruit for dipping.

▶ SERVES 6

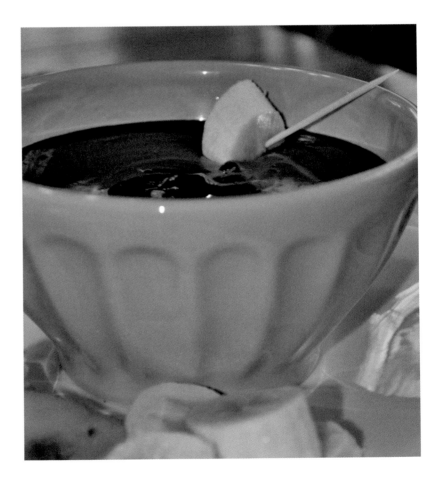

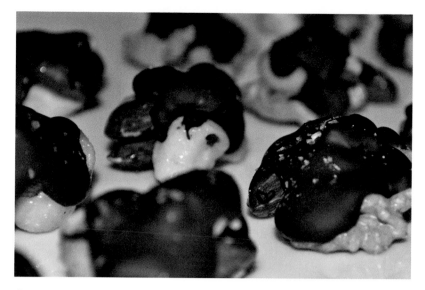

1 cup whole almonds

½ cup quartered walnuts

½ cup halved macadamia nuts

2 teaspoons blackstrap molasses

1 teaspoon agave

½ cup chocolate chips

1 teaspoon large-grain sea salt

1. Preheat oven to 350 degrees.

2. Place almonds, walnuts, and macadamia nuts in a medium bowl, and toss to combine.

3. In a small saucepan, heat molasses and agave over low heat for 30 seconds, just until melted. Drizzle over nuts and toss. Very gently, spoon about 1 tablespoon of the nut clusters onto a wire cooling rack (if you do not have one, you can spoon the same amount into mini cupcake pans coated with nonstick spray). Bake for 8 to 10 minutes.

4. Remove and let cool. Once cool, place in the freezer for at least 10 minutes.

5. Melt chocolate over a double boiler. If you do not have a double boiler, place about 3 inches of water in the bottom of a small saucepan and place a glass bowl on top of the pan. Do not let the bottom of the bowl touch the water; this will prevent burning. Place the chocolate in the bowl and bring the water up to a boil. Stir until smooth and melted.

6. Remove nut clusters from the freezer and spoon melted chocolate over the top, sprinkle evenly with sea salt, and freeze for an additional 10 minutes.

7. Serve cold or room temperature. Keep in an airtight glass container for up to 1 week or freeze for 1 month.

▶ SERVES 6

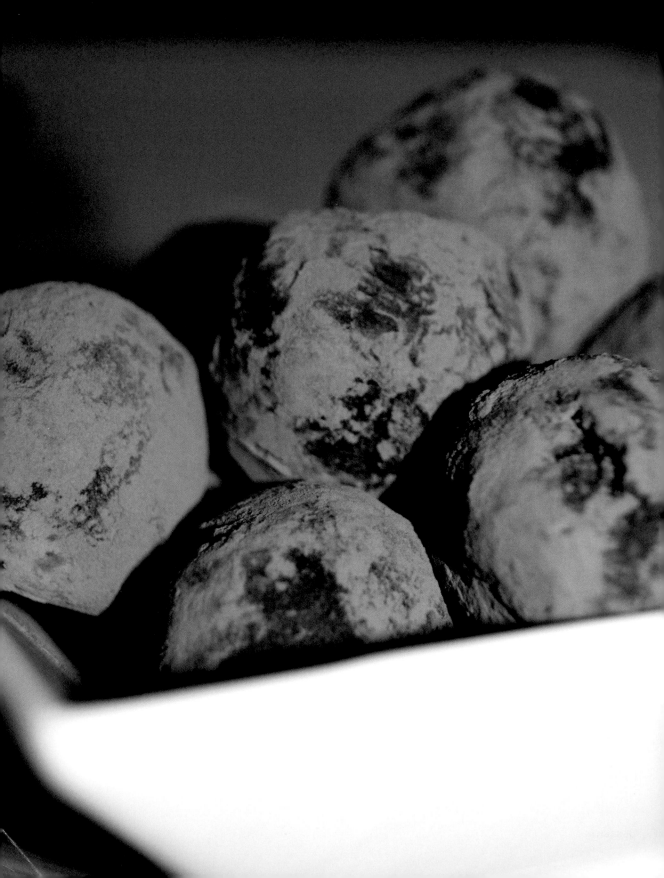

1. Shave chocolate and place in a medium bowl. Heat agave nectar, milk, and salt in a saucepan over low heat, just until warm. Pour milk mixture over chocolate, whisking continuously until mixture becomes smooth.

2. Let the mixture cool to room temperature, then cover tightly and refrigerate until chocolate is firm, about 2 to 3 hours.

3. Using a tablespoon or melon baller, scoop out truffles, roll into balls slightly smaller than a golf ball, and gently roll in cocoa powder. Refrigerate until serving.

4. Store in an airtight container in the refrigerator for up to 1 week.

▶ SERVES 6

8 ounces 100 percent dark chocolate

¼ cup ghee

⅔ cup agave nectar

½ cup (2 percent) cow's or goat's milk

⅛ teaspoon large-grain sea salt

3 tablespoons cocoa powder

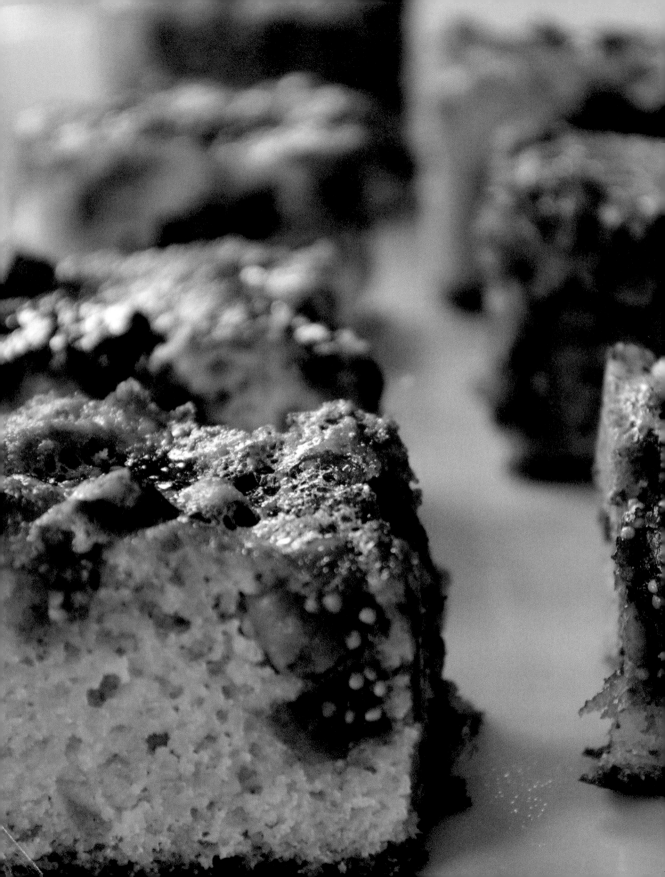

Fig Bars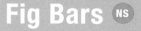

1. Preheat oven to 350 degrees. Grease a 9" × 11" baking dish with ghee, and set aside.

2. Combine flours with baking powder and sea salt in a large bowl. Mix just until combined, and set aside.

3. Whisk whole eggs with cooled ghee and add to flour mixture, mixing until smooth and free of lumps.

4. In a clean, dry glass bowl, beat egg whites until they form stiff peaks. Fold egg whites into batter, one-third at a time.

5. Pour batter into prepared baking dish and bake for about 15 minutes, until crust begins to firm.

6. While crust cooks, combine all topping ingredients in a large bowl, mixing until well combined.

7. Remove bars from oven, and spoon topping mixture evenly over par-cooked bars. Return to the oven and bake an additional 35 to 40 minutes or until a cake tester comes out clean.

8. Serve warm or room temperature.

9. Bars will stay in a cool dry place for 1 to 2 days, or in freezer for up to 1 month.

▶ SERVES 12

4 tablespoons ghee, melted and cooled, plus more for greasing

⅔ cup brown rice flour

¼ cup millet flour

¼ cup arrowroot flour

1 teaspoon baking powder

½ teaspoon sea salt

2 large eggs

2 large egg whites

topping:

½ cup fig jam

½ cup dried figs, cut into ½-inch dice

¼ cup agave

2 eggs, slightly beaten

1 egg white

2 teaspoons lemon zest

½ teaspoon ground cinnamon

⅛ teaspoon ground cloves

2 tablespoons brown rice flour

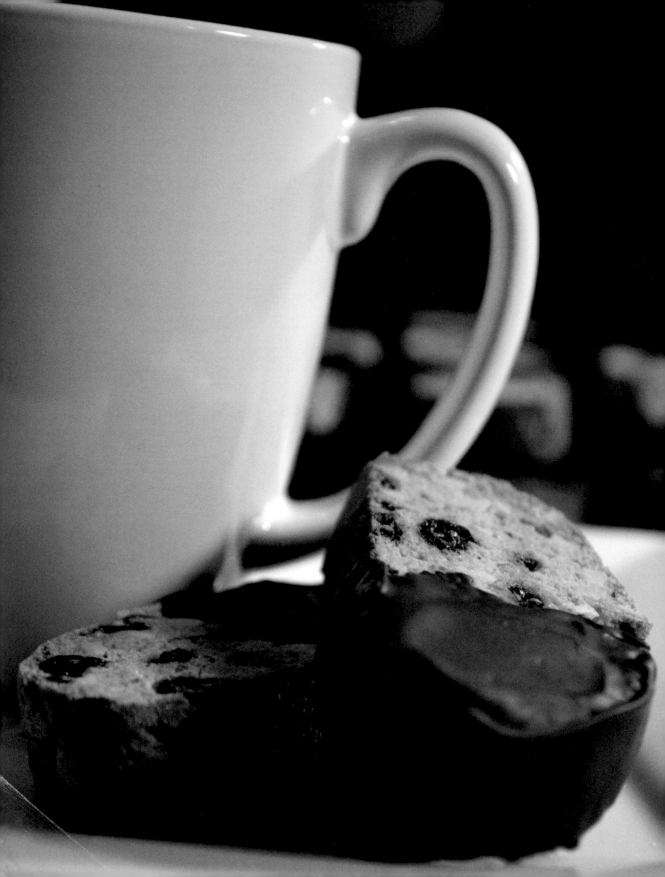

1. Preheat oven to 350 degrees. Line an 11" × 17" baking sheet with parchment paper and set aside.

2. Place cranberries in a small bowl and cover with hot water to rehydrate; let steep for 10 minutes.

3. In a large bowl, mix together flours, baking powder, salt, and almonds.

4. In a separate bowl, whisk eggs, lemon zest, agave, and apricot jam. Add egg mixture to dry ingredients, stirring just until combined. Drain cranberries, pat dry, and add to dough.

5. Gather dough into a ball and place on floured work surface. Gently roll dough with hands into a long, flat log the length of your baking sheet. Place on prepared baking sheet and bake for 30 minutes. Remove from oven and let cool 5 minutes. At this point, the cookie will have the texture of soft bread. Cut biscotti on the bias into ¾-inch slices, using a serrated knife. Place each slice flat on the baking sheet and bake for an additional 25 minutes, flipping once halfway through baking to ensure cookies are dry and crunchy all the way through.

6. Remove from oven and let cool on a drying rack. If using chocolate, heat morsels over a double boiler until melted and silky. Spoon chocolate over half of each cooled biscotti and let cool. Serve at room temperature. Store in a cool, dry place overnight or in freezer for up to 1 month.

▶ SERVES 12

¾ cup dried cranberries

1 cup amaranth flour

1½ cups brown rice flour plus more for rolling

3 teaspoons baking powder

½ teaspoon fine-grain sea salt

1 cup slivered almonds

3 large eggs

1 teaspoon lemon zest

⅓ cup agave

⅓ cup apricot jam

½ cup allergy-free chocolate chips (optional)

Chocolate Chip Cookies NS

½ cup spelt flour

½ cup oat flour

1 teaspoon sea salt

½ teaspoons baking powder

½ teaspoon baking soda

½ cup ghee, softened

½ cup agave

1 tablespoon molasses

1 teaspoon vanilla

½ cup allergy-free chocolate chips

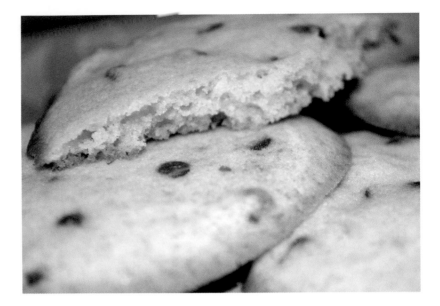

1. Preheat oven to 350 degrees. Line a 15" × 10" baking sheet with parchment paper and set aside.

2. In a large bowl, mix flours with salt, baking powder, and baking soda, and set aside.

3. In a separate bowl, beat ghee with agave, molasses, and vanilla until smooth and creamy.

4. Add ghee mixture to flour mixture and stir just until combined and free of lumps. Stir in chocolate chips. Drop dough by tablespoon 2 inches apart on prepared baking sheet.

5. Bake 12 minutes in the center rack of the oven until cookies have golden edges. Let cool on a wire rack or eat warm.

6. Cookies stay in a cool, dry place for 1 to 2 days or in the freezer up to 1 month.

▶ SERVES 12

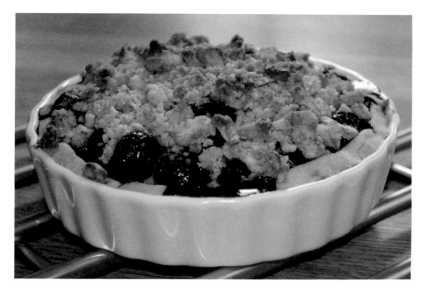

1. Preheat oven to 350 degrees.

2. Combine spelt flour and salt in a large bowl. Cut cold ghee into small pieces and add to flour mixture. Using a crossing motion with two butter knives or a pastry cutter, incorporate butter into the flour until the mixture resembles coarse corn meal. Add water, 1 tablespoon at a time, until the dough comes together but is not sticky. Gather dough in your hands and knead until it becomes smooth and pliable but small pieces of ghee should still be visible. Cover dough with plastic wrap and refrigerate 1 hour.

3. Roll dough out on a floured surface until 12 inches in diameter and approximately ⅛-inch thick. Place dough into a 9-inch pie plate, gently press into the pan, and pinch edges between two fingers to create crimped edges.

4. In a large bowl, stir together all filling ingredients just until combined, and spoon into pie crust. Set aside.

5. Combine walnuts and spelt flour in a large bowl. Use your fingers to incorporate ghee into the dough. Stir in agave and sprinkle on top of blueberry filling.

6. Bake for 25 to 30 minutes.

► SERVES 4

crust:

1 cup spelt flour plus more for rolling

¼ teaspoon sea salt

4 tablespoons ghee, chilled

4–5 tablespoons ice-cold water

filling:

1 teaspoon lemon zest

¼ teaspoon sea salt

¼ teaspoon cinnamon

⅓ cup agave

¼ teaspoon ginger

2 cups (fresh or frozen) blueberries

topping:

¼ cup finely chopped walnuts

¼ cup spelt flour

2 tablespoons ghee

1 tablespoon agave

Peach, Acai, and Cinnamon Charlotte NS

1 teaspoon ghee

1 teaspoon light olive oil

2 cups (fresh or frozen) diced peaches

¼ cup dried acai berries*

¼ cup dry toasted walnuts

3 eggs

1 tablespoon (2 percent) cow's or goat's milk

½ teaspoon cinnamon

8 slices spelt bread

1. Preheat oven to 350 degrees.

2. Heat ghee and olive oil in a skillet over medium heat. Add peaches, acai berries, and walnuts, and cook 5 minutes. Remove from heat and set aside.

3. Whisk eggs, milk, and cinnamon in a large, flat-bottomed bowl, and set aside.

4. Trim slices of bread to fit the bottom and sides of 2 (12-oz.) ramekins. Dunk bread slices in the egg wash as if making French toast. Line the bottom and edges of ramekins with the egg-soaked bread. Leave two slices of bread for the top.

5. Spoon peach mixture into the ramekins and top each with a final piece of bread.

6. Bake for 35 minutes or until golden brown.

*If you cannot find acai berries, dried cranberries can be substituted.

▶ SERVES 2

featured ingredient

acai

Acai, a tiny berry that is deep purple in color and only about an inch long, is cultivated from an acai palm tree in Central and South America. Like other berries, acai is rich in antioxidants and flavor.

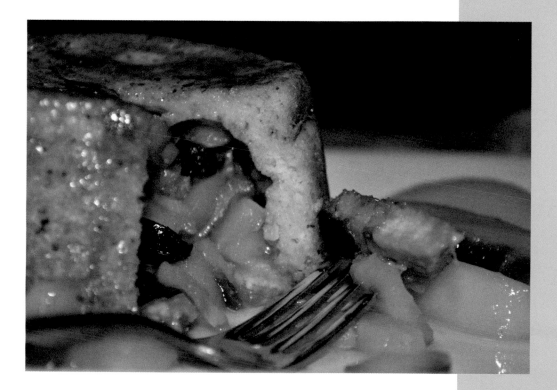

Carrot-Pineapple Cake with Chocolate Frosting NS

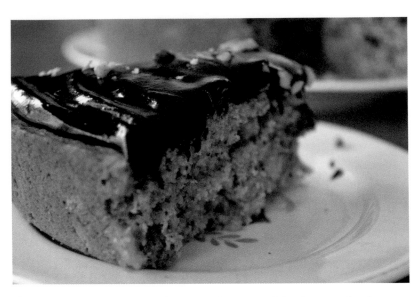

1 cup shredded carrot

¾ cup diced pineapple

1 cup brown rice flour

1 cup millet flour

¼ cup arrowroot starch

3 teaspoons baking powder

1 teaspoon salt

½ teaspoon cinnamon

2 large egg yolks

1 cup finely chopped walnuts

3 tablespoons ghee (melted and cooled) plus more for greasing

½ cup agave

4 large egg whites

frosting:

½ cup (2 percent) cow's or goat's milk

4 tablespoons agave

1 teaspoon ground cinnamon

½ teaspoon ground ginger

3 ounces 100 percent dark chocolate, grated

2 tablespoons ghee

2 tablespoons cocoa powder

¼ cup chopped walnuts, for garnish

1. Preheat oven to 350 degrees. Grease a 9-inch-round cake pan with ghee, and set aside.

2. Place shredded carrot and diced pineapple on a paper towel to absorb excess liquid.

3. In a large bowl, combine flours, arrowroot starch, baking powder, salt, and cinnamon.

4. In a separate bowl, whisk together egg yolks, pineapple, carrots, walnuts, ghee, and agave. Add to dry ingredients, stirring to combine.

5. In a dry, glass bowl, beat egg whites until they form stiff peaks. Fold egg whites into batter one-third at a time. Pour into prepared cake pan.

6. Bake 35 to 40 minutes.

7. In the meantime, heat milk and agave in a small saucepan over low heat with cinnamon and ginger for 2 to 3 minutes. Place grated chocolate in a bowl with ghee. Pour milk mixture over chocolate and whisk until smooth. Let cool completely. Add cocoa powder and stir until mixture thickens.

8. Frost cake, and sprinkle with walnuts for garnish. Serve same day for best results, or store in a cool, dry place overnight or in the freezer for up to 1 month.

▶ SERVES 8

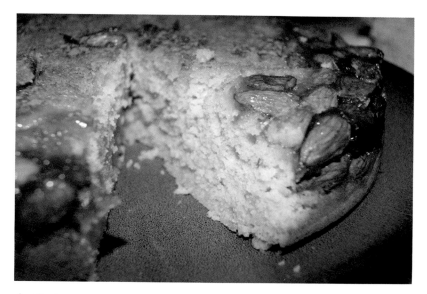

Upside-Down Almond Cake with Apricot Glaze

1. Preheat oven to 350 degrees. Grease a 9-inch-round cake pan, line with parchment paper, and set aside.

2. In a large bowl, whisk together flours, almond meal, baking powder, and salt. Set aside.

3. In a dry, glass bowl, beat egg whites with a hand mixer until they form stiff peaks, and set aside.

4. Mix remaining ingredients in a small bowl and add to dry mixture. Stir just until combined. Fold egg whites into batter, one-third at a time.

5. Scatter almonds evenly on the bottom of the cake pan. In a small saucepan, warm honey and apricot jam for 30 seconds, creating a glaze. Slowly pour evenly over almonds in the bottom of the cake pan. Pour batter over almonds and glaze and bake for 40 minutes, or until a cake tester comes out clean.

▶ SERVES 8

1 cup brown rice flour

½ cup millet flour

½ cup finely ground almond meal

2 teaspoons baking powder

½ teaspoon fine-grain sea salt

½ teaspoon lemon zest

4 large egg whites

2 large egg yolks

½ cup agave

2 tablespoons honey (NS substitute agave)

6 tablespoons ghee, softened

5 tablespoons (2 percent) cow's or goat's milk

topping:

1 cup whole almonds

2 tablespoons honey (NS substitute agave)

¼ cup sugar-free apricot jam

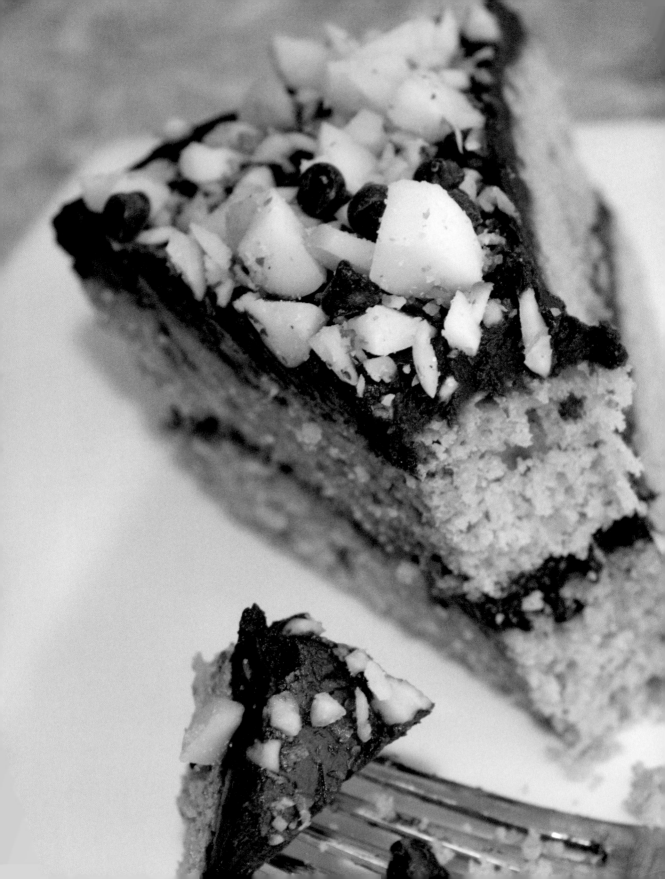

Matcha Cake with Chocolate Frosting

1. Preheat oven to 350 degrees. Grease two 9-inch-round cake pans with 1 tablespoon ghee, and set aside.

2. In a large bowl, combine dry ingredients and mix well. Set aside.

3. In a separate bowl, whisk together lemon zest, agave, ghee, eggs, egg yolk, and milk. Set aside.

4. Place egg whites in a dry glass, copper, or metal bowl and beat on high until stiff peaks form.

5. Add wet mixture to dry mixture, and stir until well combined and lump-free. Add egg whites, one-third at a time, folding gently into batter after each addition.

6. Divide batter evenly between prepared cake pans. Bake on middle oven rack for 25 minutes, until cake is firm and cake tester comes out clean. Let cool in cake pans for 10 minutes, and remove to cool fully on wire cooling racks.

7. Heat milk and agave in a small saucepan over low heat for 2 to 3 minutes. Place grated chocolate in a bowl with ghee. Pour hot milk over chocolate and stir until smooth. Let cool completely. Add cocoa powder, and stir until mixture thickens.

8. Spread slightly less than half the frosting on the first layer of cake, top with the second layer, and use an offset spatula to spread remaining frosting over the top of the second tier of cake. Sprinkle with toasted macadamia nuts and chocolate morsels.

▶ SERVES 8

1 tablespoon matcha powder

1½ cups brown rice flour

1 cup millet flour

3 teaspoons baking powder

½ teaspoon fine-grain sea salt

¼ teaspoon ground cloves

1 teaspoon lemon zest

½ cup agave

4 tablespoons ghee, melted and cooled plus 1 tablespoon for greasing

2 large eggs

1 egg yolk

⅓ cup (2 percent) cow's or goat's milk

3 large egg whites

frosting:

½ cup (2 percent) cow's or goat's milk

4 tablespoons agave

3 ounces 100 percent dark chocolate, grated

2 tablespoons ghee

2 tablespoons cocoa powder

⅔ cup chopped, toasted macadamia nuts

¼ cup allergy-free chocolate morsels

Creamy Berry Ricotta ⓝⓢ

16 ounces organic, part-skim ricotta cheese

¼ teaspoon cinnamon

1 teaspoon lemon zest

2 teaspoons agave

¼ teaspoon sea salt

½ cup fresh figs, quartered

¾ cup blueberries

¼ cup strawberries

1. In a medium-size bowl, stir together ricotta cheese, cinnamon, lemon zest, agave, and sea salt.

2. Use figs, blueberries, and strawberries to dip or stir into ricotta mixture.

▶ SERVES 4

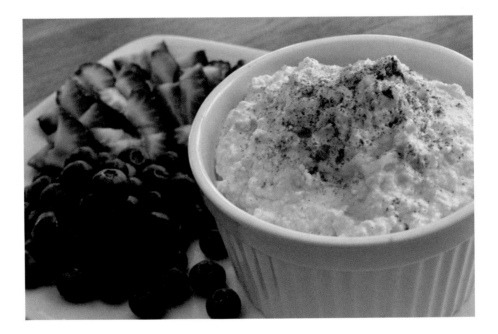

Ginger Rice Pudding

1. In a medium saucepan, bring rice, sea salt, and 2 cups milk to a boil. Reduce heat, cover, and simmer for about 45 to 50 minutes, until rice will has absorbed all the liquid in the pan.

2. In a small saucepan, heat remaining 1½ cups milk with ginger, cardamom, if using, and cinnamon over medium heat until warm, about 4 to 6 minutes.

3. In a small bowl, whisk together egg yolks, flour, molasses, and maple syrup. Temper the egg mixture by adding a ladle of the warm milk to the eggs very slowly and whisking continuously. Once the eggs have been warmed, add the mixture into the warmed milk and whisk over medium heat until the mixture is thick, 5-6 minutes, until consistency resembles yogurt. Remove from heat and set aside.

4. When rice is cooked, add pineapple and milk mixture. Let cook an additional 3 to 5 minutes over low heat, stirring continuously.

5. Rice pudding will be thick and creamy. Serve warm.

▶ SERVES 4

1 cup long-grain brown rice

½ teaspoon sea salt

3½ cups (2 percent) cow's or goat's milk, divided

1 tablespoon fresh ginger, grated

⅛ teaspoon ground cardamom (optional)

¼ teaspoon ground cinnamon

2 large egg yolks

2 tablespoons brown rice flour

1 tablespoon blackstrap molasses

1 tablespoon maple syrup (NS substitute agave)

½ cup diced, dried pineapple (no sugar added)

Millet Crêpes with Raspberry Chutney and Chocolate Syrup NS

crêpes:

¾ cups millet flour

¼ cup spelt flour

½ teaspoon sea salt

½ teaspoon cinnamon

1¼ cups (2 percent) cow's or goat's milk

1 large egg

1 tablespoon plus 1 teaspoon ghee, melted and cooled

chutney:

1 teaspoon ghee

1 Bosc pear, diced

1 teaspoon lemon zest

½ teaspoon grated fresh ginger

¼ cup no sugar added apricot jam

1 cup halved fresh raspberries*

Chocolate Syrup*

1. Combine flours, salt, cinnamon, milk, egg, and 1 tablespoon ghee in a blender and pulse until smooth and combined. Batter will be very thin. Let rest in the refrigerator for 1 hour.

2. While batter rests, heat ghee in a medium skillet over medium heat. Sauté pear for 3 to 4 minutes, or until slightly browned and tender. Add lemon zest, ginger, and apricot jam, and cook 30 seconds. Remove from heat and toss with fresh raspberries.

3. Preheat oven to 200 degrees.

4. Heat a large skillet over medium heat. When the pan is hot, melt 1 teaspoon of ghee and brush evenly across the bottom of the pan. Using a ¼-cup measure, scoop batter into pan and quickly turn in circular motions to spread the batter into a very thin layer. Let cook 1 minute or until the batter firms and edges lift slightly off the pan. Use an offset spatula to flip and cook 1 minute. Repeat with remaining batter. Stack finished crêpes in a slightly moist kitchen towel and keep in the oven until ready to serve.

5. To serve, place a spoonful of chutney down the center of a crêpe, and roll up like a soft taco. Drizzle with Chocolate Syrup and serve warm.

*See Chocolate Syrup NS recipe (page 218).

▶ SERVES 4

tip: Cranberries can be substituted for raspberries. Just cook with 1 tablespoon agave.

Stocks, Condiments, and Sauces

Honey-Mustard Dressing

2 tablespoons spicy mustard

¼ cup extra virgin olive oil

1 tablespoon honey (NS substitute agave)

Sea salt, to taste

1. Whisk all ingredients together in a small bowl, or pour ingredients in a resealable glass jar and shake vigorously to combine. Season with sea salt, to taste.

2. Store salad dressing in a glass jar or dispenser in the refrigerator for up to 1 week. Recipe can be doubled so that you have it ready to go all week.

KO's Ketchup NS

2 tablespoons finely chopped onion

1 teaspoon olive oil

½ cup organic tomato paste

1 tablespoon agave

2 tablespoons apple juice

½ teaspoon salt

1 tablespoon lemon juice

1 teaspoon blackstrap molasses

1. Heat olive oil in a small skillet over medium heat and sauté onion for 3 to 4 minutes. Add remaining ingredients, and simmer for 4 minutes. Spoon into a bowl or glass jar and cool. Store in the refrigerator, and use as ketchup substitute.

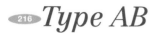

Citus Dressing NS

1. Whisk all ingredients together in a small bowl, or pour ingredients in a resealable glass jar and shake vigorously to combine. Season with sea salt, to taste.

2. Store salad dressing in a glass jar or dispenser in the refrigerator for up to 1 week. Recipe can be doubled so that you have it ready to go all week.

¼ cup extra virgin olive oil

Juice of 1 lemon

Juice of 1 lime

1 tablespoon finely chopped cilantro

1 teaspoon agave

Sea salt, to taste

Herb Dressing NS

1. Whisk all ingredients together in a small bowl, or pour ingredients in a resealable glass jar and shake vigorously to combine. Season with sea salt, to taste.

2. Store salad dressing in a glass jar or dispenser in the refrigerator for up to 1 week. Recipe can be doubled so that you have it ready to go all week.

¼ cup finely chopped fresh basil

2 tablespoons finely chopped fresh parsley

2 tablespoons finely chopped fresh chives

2 small cloves garlic, minced

½ cup extra virgin olive oil

⅔ cup fresh-squeezed lemon juice

Sea salt, to taste

Carrot-Ginger Dressing NS

1 tablespoon fresh carrot juice

2 medium carrots

1 tablespoon olive oil

1 (1-inch) piece ginger, peeled

Sea salt, to taste

1. In the food processor, pulse carrot juice, carrots, olive oil, and ginger until smooth. If the mixture is too thick, add water, 1 table-spoon at a time.

2. Season with sea salt, to taste, and store in a glass container or dispenser in the refrigerator for up to 1 week.

Chocolate Syrup NS

1 cup agave

2 tablespoons cocoa powder

1. Whisk agave and cocoa powder vigorously in a bowl to incorporate. Use to drizzle over pancakes or fruit, or to add a special treat to smoothies.

2. Store in a cool, dry place for up to 2 weeks.

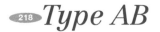

Cinnamon Syrup

1. Melt ghee in a saucepan over medium-low heat. Add agave and cinnamon, whisking until smooth and combined. Remove from heat and let cool completely.

2. Store in a clean, glass dispenser or container in the refrigerator for up to 2 weeks.

2 teaspoons ghee
1 cup agave
2 teaspoons cinnamon

Turkey Stock

4 pounds turkey thighs and breast

3 large carrots, peeled and diced

1 celery root, peeled and diced

2 cloves garlic, peeled

1 Vidalia onion, chopped

4 quarts water

2 teaspoons sea salt

3 sprigs fresh thyme

3 sprigs fresh rosemary

5 sprigs parsley

2 bay leaves

1. Bring all ingredients to a gentle boil in a large stockpot. As the stock boils, use a large spoon to skim foam and impurities off the top and discard.

2. Reduce heat and simmer, 3 hours. Remove ingredients from stock and strain into a clean bowl or pot.

3. Let stock cool (no longer than 4 hours). Store in glass containers in the refrigerator for up to 3 days or in the freezer for 2 months.

4. Turkey meat can be used for salad, casseroles, or to add to your soup. Pick the meat off the bones, cool it, and refrigerate for another use.

Vegetable Stock NS

1. Heat olive oil in a large stockpot over medium heat. Add onion, celery root, parsnips, carrots, and fennel, and cook for 8 to 10 minutes. Add water and remaining ingredients and bring to a boil. Cover, reduce heat to low, and cook for 30 minutes. (Vegetable stock has a quick cooking time because vegetables give up their flavor quickly, as opposed to meats and bones.)

2. Strain stock into a clean pot and store in the refrigerator for 3 to 5 days or in the freezer for 2 to 3 months.

2 teaspoons olive oil

2 onions, chopped

1 celery root, peeled and chopped

1 cup parsnips, chopped

1 cup carrots, chopped

2 bulbs fennel, chopped

4 quarts water

3 tomatoes, halved

3 bay leaves

1 clove garlic, peeled

5 sprigs parsley

5 sprigs thyme

2 teaspoons sea salt

Basic Bread Crumbs

4 slices spelt or oat
bread

1. Toast slices of bread and let cool. Pulse cooled toast in a food
processor to form coarse crumbs. To add flavor, add dried herbs
such as parsley, rosemary, thyme, sage, and/or basil.

Useful Tools

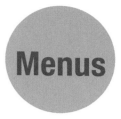

Substitutions

An integral part of acclimating to your new diet is being able to fill in the void created by your *Best Avoided* list. Below is a list of substitutions to help you along the way. A number of these are not direct substitutions, but you will see from recipes in this book how they are adapted to work in place of items on your *Best Avoided* list.

BREAD—The beauty about having blood Type AB is that there are many bread options out there for you. Be certain, however, to read the labels of bread you buy in the store. A bread may carry the claim of being "whole grain oat bread" but will contain white flour or some other ingredient that is on your *Avoid* list. We always recommend variety in a healthy diet, so even if you find great oat bread, try a spelt, rye, or sprouted wheat version to mix things up and diversify your nutritional intake.

PASTA—The best pasta you can get is made from either spelt or brown rice. Similar to breads, however, many varieties contain corn or wheat flour so be sure to read the label.

BUTTER—This may be one of those things that is difficult to let go of. A terrific alternative, however, is ghee, which is simply clarified butter. When butter is heated, it separates and the lactose comes to the top and the fat remains on the bottom. When the lactose is removed, what remains is called ghee. Use it just like butter, to spread on toast or add to rice or vegetables. Ghee is never salted, so when you are spreading it on toast you might want to add a touch of sea salt.

FLOUR—The best flours for baking are a combination for texture and taste. In this book we try to incorporate highly *Beneficial* flours.

Although those following the Type AB diet can have whole wheat, combinations such as spelt and oat, or brown rice and millet, are the most *Beneficial* grains. Whole wheat can have a very earthy taste and hearty texture, whereas spelt and oat lend more of a tender softness that seems to be more appealing for most people.

Two great everyday baking mixes for Type AB are:

> 2 parts spelt flour (⅔ cup for one batch)
> 1 part oat flour (⅓ cup for one batch)
> Add 2 teaspoons baking powder and ½ teaspoon sea salt to each batch.

or:

> 1 part brown rice flour (⅓ cup for one batch)
> 1 part millet flour (⅓ cup for one batch)
> 1 part arrowroot starch (⅓ cup for one batch)
> Add 2 teaspoons baking powder and ½ teaspoon sea salt to each batch.

Menu Planning

The following are suggestions to show you how to put the recipes in this book together to create weekly menus for you and your family. They are arranged in a way to keep a balanced diet, but feel free to mix and match as you see fit. If you plan to follow the menu exactly, read it thoroughly ahead of time so you can see where you would need to buy a little extra to account for leftovers, and where it would be practical to plan/prep ahead. The purpose of menu planning is to make life as easy as possible by utilizing leftovers and planning more involved meals for weekends.

In addition to the list below, make sure you are drinking a minimum of six (8-oz.) glasses of water per day to stay properly hydrated.

MENU PLANNING TIPS:

- If you are working full-time or have difficulty preparing meals during the week, use time on the weekend to prepare snacks and a few meals for the week by prewashing vegetables and lettuce. This will significantly cut down on weekday duties. A few foods that stay well and that I always have on hand are: Flax Crackers,

Blackstrap-Cherry Granola, Spicy Rosemary-Nut Clusters, and occasionally a Unibar® Protein Bar.

- If you don't like leftovers, it's time to start liking them. Leftovers are the most delightful time-savers you could imagine. Pair them with a fresh salad or toss in a soup, and they will become your best friend, too.

- When making something like bruschetta, double the topping recipe and reserve leftovers in a sealable glass container in the refrigerator for up to 1 week. That way, you make the dish once and it can be used as many times as you want it.

- When baking breads, muffins, or even sweet treats, freeze leftovers in sealable glass containers to keep them fresh. If, for example, you have Pumpkin Muffins in the freezer, you can pop them in the oven or toaster oven at 200 degrees for 10 to 15 minutes and they will be perfectly toasty and ready to eat. Frozen chocolate chip cookies are also delicious and don't require defrosting . . . just one of the great things about gluten-free flour.

Four-Week Meal Planner

Week 1

Sunday

BREAKFAST: Wild-Rice Waffles NS with sliced banana and raw walnuts

LUNCH: Ratatouille NS

SNACK: Cucumber slices with Curried Egg Salad NS

DINNER: Turkey Chili NS

Monday

BREAKFAST: Blackstrap-Cherry Granola NS, rice cereal, yogurt with fresh blueberries, and green tea

LUNCH: Leftover Turkey Chili NS with mixed greens salad dressed with lemon and olive oil

SNACK: Pear and Apple Chips NS and Spicy Rosemary-Nut Clusters

DINNER: Lemon-Ginger Salmon with Brown Rice Salad NS

Tuesday

BREAKFAST: Scrambled eggs with Blueberry-Walnut Muffins and green tea

LUNCH: Raw Kale Salad with Zesty Lime Dressing NS and leftover Lemon-Ginger Salmon

SNACK: Flax Crackers NS and Heirloom Tomato and Eggplant Salsa

DINNER: Crispy-Coated Turkey Tenderloins with Apricot Dipping Sauce NS and Ratatouille NS

Wednesday

BREAKFAST: Homemade Turkey Breakfast Sausage NS with sliced pineapple and green tea

LUNCH: Raw Kale Salad with Zesty Lime Dressing NS and leftover Crispy-Coated Turkey Tenderloins with Apricot Dipping Sauce NS

SNACK: Pear and Apple Chips NS and Spicy Rosemary-Nut Clusters

DINNER: Grilled Radicchio and Walnut-Spinach Pesto NS

Thursday

BREAKFAST: Blueberry-Walnut Muffins with leftover Homemade Turkey Breakfast Sausage NS and green tea

LUNCH: Greens and Beans Salad with feta cheese

SNACK: Protein Blend™ Powder—Type B/AB drink

DINNER: Tangy Pineapple and Tempeh Kabobs NS with Roasted Autumn Roots NS

Friday

BREAKFAST: Quinoa Muesli NS, banana slices, blueberries, and green tea

LUNCH: Leftover Greens and Beans Salad with leftover Tangy Pineapple and Tempeh Kabobs NS

SNACK: Carob–Walnut Butter–Stuffed Figs NS

DINNER: Roasted Tomato and Broccoli Mac and Cheese NS and Garlic-Creamed Collards and Spinach NS

Saturday

BREAKFAST: Broccoli-Feta Frittata NS with green tea and pineapple

LUNCH: ½ Bacon Grilled Cheese NS with Melted Mozzarella–Onion Soup NS

SNACK: Peanut Butter Rice Cakes with Mini Chips

DINNER: Seafood Paella NS

Week 2

Sunday

BREAKFAST: Cherry Scones NS with peanut butter and green tea

LUNCH: Pinto Bean Stew NS

SNACK: Grilled Pineapple with Cinnamon Syrup

DINNER: Moroccan Lamb Tagine NS

Monday

BREAKFAST: Breakfast Egg Salad NS

LUNCH: Mint and Cherry Tomato Tabbouleh with leftover Moroccan Lamb Tagine NS

SNACK: Homemade Applesauce

DINNER: Shredded Turkey Bake NS

Tuesday

BREAKFAST: Quinoa Muesli NS with sliced bananas and fresh blueberries

LUNCH: Leftover Shredded Turkey Bake NS with mixed greens dressed in olive oil and lemon

SNACK: Grilled Pineapple with Cinnamon Syrup

DINNER: Pasta Carbonara with Crispy Kale NS

Wednesday

BREAKFAST: Turkey Bacon–Spinach Squares NS with sliced pineapple and green tea

LUNCH: Leftover Pasta Carbonara with Crispy Kale NS

SNACK: Toasty Pizza Bites NS

DINNER: Lamb Steaks in a Wild-Mushroom Sauce NS

Thursday

BREAKFAST: Broccoli-Feta Frittata NS with green tea

LUNCH: Navy Bean Hummus and Feta Sandwich NS

SNACK: Homemade Applesauce

DINNER: Turkey Meat Loaf with Spicy Collards NS and Baked Beans

Friday

BREAKFAST: Granola–Nut Butter Fruit Slices NS with green tea

LUNCH: Leftover Turkey Meat Loaf sandwiches
SNACK: Protein Blend™ Powder—Type B/AB drink
DINNER: Spicy Seafood Stew

Saturday

BREAKFAST: Spelt Pancakes NS with scrambled eggs and green tea
LUNCH: Salmon-Filled Radicchio Cups
SNACK: Crispy Spring Vegetable Cakes NS
DINNER: Sweet Potato Gnocchi with Basil-Cranberry Sauce NS with mozzarella cheese

Week 3

Sunday

BREAKFAST: Pear-Rosemary Bread NS with poached egg and green tea
LUNCH: Fish Fillet Sandwich
SNACK: Crudités and Creamy Goat Cheese Dip NS
DINNER: Turkey Mole Drumsticks with Whipped Sweet Potato Soufflé NS and Broccoli and Cabbage Slaw

Monday

BREAKFAST: Creamy Almond Butter Smoothie NS and green tea
LUNCH: Leftover Turkey Mole Drumsticks and Broccoli and Cabbage Slaw
SNACK: Unibar® Protein Bar
DINNER: Salmon Soybean Cakes with Cilantro-Cream Sauce NS and Spicy Roasted Mustard Greens with Feta NS

Tuesday

BREAKFAST: Pear-Rosemary Bread NS with scrambled eggs and green tea
LUNCH: Leftover Salmon Soybean Cakes with Cilantro-Cream Sauce NS and romaine dressed in lemon and olive oil
SNACK: Marinated Mozzarella NS with Flax Crackers NS
DINNER: Slow-Cooker Butternut Squash–Lentil Stew NS with Sweet-and-Salty Brussels

Wednesday

BREAKFAST: Turkey Bacon–Spinach Squares NS and green tea

LUNCH: Leftover Slow-Cooker Butternut Squash–Lentil Stew NS

SNACK: Unibar® Protein Bar

DINNER: Broccoli Northern Bean Soup NS with Green Tea Poached Turkey Tenderloin NS

Thursday

BREAKFAST: Blackstrap-Cherry Granola NS, rice cereal, yogurt with fresh blueberries, and green tea

LUNCH: Shredded leftover Green Tea–Poached Turkey Tenderloin NS with cranberries and walnuts over spinach with olive oil and lemon

SNACK: Marinated Mozzarella NS with Flax Crackers NS

DINNER: Herb-Crusted Turkey Breast Stuffed with Shallots and Figs NS with Roasted Pumpkin with Fried Sage NS

Friday

BREAKFAST: Homemade Turkey Breakfast Sausage NS with sliced pineapple and green tea

LUNCH: Leftover Herb-Crusted Turkey Breast Stuffed with Shallots and Figs NS over Raw Kale Salad with Zesty Lime Dressing NS

SNACK: Unibar® Protein Bar

DINNER: Turkey Sausage–Zucchini Boats with Wild-Grain Soup with Sun-Dried Tomato Pesto NS

Saturday

BREAKFAST: Kale and Zucchini Soufflé NS and green tea

LUNCH: Crunchy Green Bean and Beet Spring Rolls with Sweet Cherry Dip NS

SNACK: Farmer Cheese and Beet-Endive Cups NS

DINNER: Spring Pesto Pasta NS with grilled salmon

Week 4

Sunday

BREAKFAST: Savory Herb and Cheese Bread Pudding NS

Type AB 231

LUNCH: Navy Bean Hummus and Feta Sandwich NS

SNACK: Fruit Salad with Mint-Lime Dressing NS

DINNER: Sweet Potato Shepherd's Pie NS with Roasted Tomato and Broccoli Mac and Cheese NS

Monday

BREAKFAST: Maple-Sausage Scramble and green tea

LUNCH: Leftover Sweet Potato Shepherd's Pie NS

SNACK: Roasted Cauliflower Bruschetta NS

DINNER: Noodles with Poached Salmon and Basil Cream NS and Roasted Escarole NS

Tuesday

BREAKFAST: Pumpkin Muffins with Carob Drizzle NS with peanut butter and green tea

LUNCH: Baked Falafel NS with Roasted Tomato Greek Salad NS

SNACK: Fruit Salad with Mint-Lime Dressing NS

DINNER: Lentil Burgers and Asparagus with Crispy Walnut Bacon

Wednesday

BREAKFAST: Granola–Nut Butter Fruit Slices with Tropical Kale Smoothie NS and green tea

LUNCH: Leftover Asparagus with Crispy Walnut Bacon wrapped in Boston Bibb lettuce with feta cheese

SNACK: Crudités and Creamy Goat Cheese Dip NS

DINNER: Ginger-Tofu Stir-Fry NS with Carrot-Ginger Soup NS

Thursday

BREAKFAST: Breakfast Egg Salad NS with green tea

LUNCH: Leftover Carrot-Ginger Soup NS and ½ Bacon Grilled Cheese NS

SNACK: Roasted Cauliflower Bruschetta NS

DINNER: Pasta Carbonara with Crispy Kale NS with Greens and Beans Salad

Friday

BREAKFAST: Pumpkin Muffins with Carob Drizzle NS with peanut butter and green tea

LUNCH: Leftover Greens and Beans Salad with walnuts and fresh mozzarella cheese

SNACK: Crudités and Creamy Goat Cheese Dip NS

DINNER: Fish Tacos with Bean and Crunchy Fennel Slaw NS

Saturday

BREAKFAST: Cinnamon-Oat Crêpes NS and green tea

LUNCH: Melted Mozzarella–Onion Soup NS

SNACK: Baked Grapefruit

DINNER: Turkey Pot Pie with Crunchy Topping

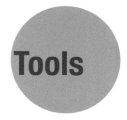

Tools

YOU CAN FIND the following helpful tools on our Personalized Living page at http://www.4yourtype.com/cookbooks.asp. From there, you will be able to download these PDFs and print them from your computer:

- Food Journal
  Keep track of every meal with this handy log.

- Tracking Your Progress
  This is an additional log to help you focus on your goals.

- Shopping List
  Make your shopping trip easy with this list of *Beneficial* foods for your type.

TYPE AB SHOPPING LIST:

Produce

Beets	Kale	Grapefruit
Broccoli	Parsnips	Pineapple
Cauliflower	Sweet potato	Watermelon
Eggplant	Figs	
Garlic	Grapes	

Baking

Agave	Molasses	Soy flour
Baking powder	Oat flour	Spelt flour
Brown rice flour	Sea salt	

Dairy

Cottage cheese	Ghee	Goat cheese
Eggs	Goat's milk	Ricotta
Feta cheese	Mozzarella cheese	Yogurt

Meat/Seafood

Cod	Red snapper	Turkey
Lamb	Salmon	
Mahimahi	Tuna	

Miscellaneous

Olive oil	Soybeans	Parsley
Almonds	Tempeh	Curry
Peanuts	Tofu	Chamomile tea
Peanut butter	Oat bread	Ginger tea
Walnuts	Spelt bread	Green tea
Lentils	Sprouted wheat	Red wine
Navy beans	bread	

Please note: This shopping list only highlights the most frequently used *Beneficial* and some *Neutral* foods for Type AB. For a complete list of *Beneficial, Neutral,* and *Avoid,* please reference *Eat Right 4 Your Type,* the *Blood Type AB Food, Beverage, and Supplement Lists,* or consult your SWAMI personalized nutrition report if you have one.

Time to Think Green

MICHEL NISCHAN IS a sustainable chef, cookbook author, and connoisseur of local, healthy food. He wrote in one of his books, *Sustainably Delicious: Making the World a Better Place, One Recipe at a Time*, "Where there is flavor, there are nutrients, and where there are nutrients, there is health." It is well known by chefs around the globe that the best food comes from the freshest ingredients, and nothing is fresher than a tomato grown in your own backyard or at the local farm. When you meander through your local farmers market and browse fruits and vegetables picked at their peak of freshness, the smells, touch, and tastes become infinitely more vibrant than a similar stroll through the supermarket. If you start any meal with fresh, local, whole-food ingredients, almost anything you make will be the best-tasting food and the best for your health.

Here are a few highlights on buying organic, avoiding toxins in your kitchen, and shopping for the freshest fruits and vegetables.

Quick Review of the Terms

Whenever possible, buy organic food and grass-fed beef. Why? Conventional fruits and vegetables are sprayed with harmful chemicals such as herbicides, pesticides, and insecticides. The chemicals used in these substances can disrupt hormones, and potentially cause cancer, allergies, asthma, and other health issues. Conventionally raised meat, dairy, and poultry exist in poor conditions and are fed for the purpose of fast weight gain, which is taxing to their health. As a result, animals are given antibiotics, which end up in the meat you buy at the grocery store. In addition, some animals are put on hormones to bulk up their bodies, making their meat artificially larger and, therefore, more desirable to consumers' eyes. Eating turkey is a terrific source of healing food for Type ABs, but if the meat is contaminated with hormones and antibiotics and causes unnecessary disruptions to your system, the goodness is essentially negated.

 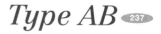

Here are a few definitions to sort out some of the confusion:

100 Percent USDA Certified Organic—This means that the product you purchase must contain only organic ingredients, minus water and salt. Knowing the abbreviation USDA is an easy way to identify foods that are 100 percent certified organic.

Organic—Products must contain a minimum of 95 percent organic ingredients. Each ingredient within the product that is organic must also be labeled as such.

Made with Organic Ingredients—Indicates that 70 percent or more organic ingredients are contained in the product. The word *organic* cannot be prominently displayed on these products.

Natural—The product contains no artificial ingredients or added color and is processed in a way that does not fundamentally alter the product.

No Hormones—This term can only be used for beef. Poultry and pork are not allowed to be raised using hormones, so the label is unnecessary.

Grass-Fed—This term applies to animals that are solely fed grass and hay.

Free-Range—This indicates that animals are allowed access to the outside. This label is tricky, however, because there are a large number of farms that keep their animals in poor conditions but allow a tiny space for "outdoor access" in order to be labeled "Free Range." Check out http://www.cornucopia.org/organic-egg-scorecard to determine if the eggs you buy are coming from humane farms.

Tips for Buying Local and Organic
Choosing Food That Is in Season

This phrase is tossed around a lot, but what is the benefit of eating in season? Taste. Obviously, it also has a significant environmental impact, but the difference between eating a fresh, off-the-vine heirloom tomato versus a genetically modified tomato from the grocery store is striking enough to convince even the harshest skeptics. Eating in season also ensures that you are rotating the kinds of vegetables in your diet, and as a result, the nutrients. There is nothing more refreshing than fresh watermelon in the summer or roasted pumpkin in the fall. Make a habit of eating only the best by choosing local, organic food that is in season.

Where to Find Fresh Food in Season?

Look for local listings indicating farm stands or farmers markets. Most farms are also happy to show you around if you want to stop by for a visit or take your children to see how food is grown and raised. A terrific resource for finding local food is: www.localharvest.org. Just fill out your city/state, and you will be provided with a listing of local and organic food happenings. Eating in season is more satisfying to the body and palate.

Local or Organic?

Sometimes we have to make the choice between eating local food or organic food, and it can be confusing. Local food is terrific because of its freshness and limited impact on the environment; it does not have to be shipped all the way from Chile to get to your table. Food that is organic, however, is grown without harmful chemicals that are detrimental to your health but that also negatively impact our environment. In an ideal world, we wouldn't have to choose between organic and pesticide-free foods, but sometimes that is the choice we are faced with as consumers. Thankfully many independent, local farms practice organic farming, which can limit the need for these choices.

Healthy Choices on a Budget?

At some point, we all have to watch what we spend on everything, including food. The number-one tip for maintaining a healthy diet on a budget is prioritizing. If you are eating right for your blood type, you will be cutting out extras like potato chips, soda, prepared dips, cookies, and most overly processed foods. This alone will start to make room in your budget for healthier alternatives. Additionally, buying food in season is far less expensive than buying those same foods out of season. For example, a pint of organic blueberries in the middle of the winter can cost up to $6.99; the same pint at the farmers market in the summer can go as low as $2.99. When stocking up on grains or nuts, be savvy and buy in bulk. Nuts contain fats that if left in your pantry could spoil quickly. Excess nuts can be stored in the freezer for several months. Buying in bulk also means you are cutting down on the cost and waste of excess packaging, which you definitely pay for.

Finally, prioritizing your organic purchases will save you a bundle. There are twelve fruits and vegetables that carry the most pesticide residue; therefore, buying these ingredients organic should take priority. (See the foods on the Dirty Dozen listed below.) If you are on a budget, don't cut out these foods entirely, simply cut back how many you buy in one trip. Try to pick one or two ingredients that you must buy organic and supplement them with produce known to carry the lowest levels of pesticides, also known as the Clean Fifteen.

Dirty Dozen/Clean Fifteen

Below is a list of the Dirty Dozen*. Try to buy these organic as often as possible to reduce your pesticide exposure.

1. Apples
2. Celery
3. Strawberries
4. Peaches
5. Spinach
6. Nectarines—imported
7. Grapes—imported
8. Sweet bell peppers (*Avoid* for AB)
9. Potatoes
10. Blueberries—domestic
11. Lettuce
12. Kale/Collard greens

Listed here are the Clean Fifteen*, a list of produce that has the smallest traces of pesticides and are therefore safest to buy in their conventional form. If it is possible, however, choosing organic is always better for yourself and the environment.

1. Onions
2. Sweet corn (*Avoid* for AB)
3. Pineapples
4. Avocado (*Avoid* for AB)
5. Asparagus
6. Sweet peas
7. Mangoes (*Avoid* for AB)
8. Eggplant
9. Cantaloupe—domestic
10. Kiwi
11. Cabbage
12. Watermelon
13. Sweet potatoes
14. Grapefruit
15. Mushrooms

*Dirty Dozen and Clean Fifteen taken from the Environmental Working Group website, www.ewg.org.

Safe Food Storage

The first question is, what is safe? As most of us are aware, there is a chemical in most plastics called BPA (Biphenol-A), which, when ingested, acts as a hormone disrupter. Studies recently conducted report that BPA negatively affects hormone levels, which can lead to obesity as well as problems with thyroid function and the risk of certain cancers.

Where Is BPA Found?

BPA is a compound found in consumer products such as plastic containers, water bottles, plastic wrap, cans, and some cartons. Plastics labeled 3, 6, or 7 for recycling purposes often contain BPA.

What Makes BPA Leach into Our Food?

Cans contain BPA in their lining. Therefore, when a can contains foods with high levels of acidity (such as tomatoes), there is a greater likelihood that BPA will seep into the food. Foods with high acidity also affect plastics,

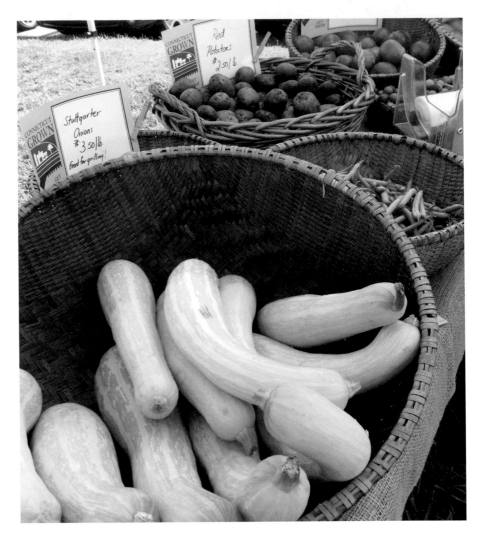

but a drastic change in the temperature of plastics (like freezing or being left in a warm car) will have the same leaching effect.

How Do I Avoid Them?

Thankfully, it is getting easier and easier to avoid BPA, mostly because the chemical is being banned by the government in most products for children. Additionally, the more we know about the harmful effects of BPA, the more demand there is in the market for products that are free of this harmful chemical. There are a many companies making available BPA-free products. A terrific alternative to canned tomatoes are products packaged by Tetra Pak; all of its packaging is BPA-free. Additionally, look for foods packaged in glass jars as opposed to cans or plastics.

What Should Be Done About Buying Food in Plastic/Cans?

The best way to purchase food is fresh, in glass, or in Tetra Pak cartons. Meats and seafood that are packaged by your butcher in plastic can be swapped out at home for further storage. If you feel inclined, however, let your butcher know you would prefer your food wrapped in paper. If enough people speak up, a change will certainly happen.

How Do I Pack Safe School Lunches?

Traditionally, kids' lunch boxes and plastic bottles contained BPA. The good news is that there are an increasing number of BPA-free options available now; you just have to look out for them. Due to recent studies about the adverse effects of BPA on health, most companies are trying to or are required by law to switch to BPA-free materials. That being said, glass containers with sealable lids are available in many different sizes and are another great alternative to plastic.

   NOTE: Get kids involved, so they start learning young. Let them help you in the process of preparing and packing their lunches. This allows them to learn about healthier nutrition. Choose fun, nontoxic snack packs for them to store their lunches.

Cleaning up the Kitchen

What's Wrong with Chemicals?

Traditional household cleaners contain chemicals such as alkylphenols, alkylphenol ethoxylates, ammonia, chlorine, and diethanolamine, just to name a few. These chemicals can cause allergies, skin irritation, asthma, and potentially much more serious health problems. Avoiding these chemicals and others in our environment is pretty much impossible, but what we can do is become aware of where they exist, and limit our exposure as much as possible. The first step is cleaning out your detergents, bleach, disinfectant sprays, or wipes along with any other cleaning products.

Is It More Expensive to Use Natural Cleaners?

If you're smart about it, it doesn't have to be. In fact, cleaning with natural products can actually be less expensive. For example, vinegar is mentioned below as a replacement to some cleaning products. A generic brand of vinegar is about $0.02/ounce, and a little definitely goes a long way.

What Are Some Household Products That Can Clean Well?

The best nontoxic cleaners are: vinegar, baking soda, lemon juice, and club soda. Vinegar is a natural disinfectant and, believe it or not, deodorizer. You can use it on floors, countertops, sinks, and any surface that needs cleaning. Baking soda mixed with water is slightly abrasive and can be used to clean stainless steel and carpets, and also acts as a fabric softener and deodorizer.

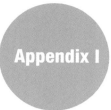

Additional Information on the Blood Type Diet

Discover Your Blood Type

It is difficult to begin a diet based on blood type if you are not aware of your own type. In Europe, blood type is something almost everyone knows, but here in the United States, unless we need a transfusion, we can go our entire lives without knowing what blood type we are. Here are several simple ways to find out your type:

Donate blood. Not only are you providing a critical service to the community, but this is a free and simple way to find out what blood type you are. To find your local donation center, visit the American Red Cross website's Give Blood page (www.redcrossblood.org).

Purchase a blood-typing test kit at D'Adamo Personalized Nutrition (www.4yourtype.com), under Books and Tests. The kit is inexpensive and simple to do in your own home.

Next time you visit your doctor for a blood workup, ask him or her to add blood type to the blood-draw protocol.

Secretor Status

In this book, we also address Secretor Status, tagging each recipe to indicate if it is appropriate for both Secretors and Non-Secretors. If you do not know your Secretor Status, you can purchase a Secretor Status Test Kit from D'Adamo Personalized Nutrition (www.4yourtype.com).

Center of Excellence in Generative Medicine

The Center of Excellence (COE) in Generative Medicine is a collaboration between Dr. Peter D'Adamo and the University of Bridgeport to create a frontiers-focused biomedical initiative without parallel in any other medical school. The COE combines patient care, clinical research, and hands-on teaching opportunities for students in UB's Health Sciences program. It is also home to Dr. Peter D'Adamo's clinical practice. For information and appointments for either private-practice patients or clinic-shift patients, please contact:

Center of Excellence in Generative Medicine
115 Broad Street
Bridgeport, CT 06604
(203) 366-0526
www.generativemedicine.org/

D'Adamo Personalized Nutrition®—North American Pharmacal, Inc.

For information on the Blood Type Diet, individualized supplements, and testing kits, please contact:
North American Pharmacal, Inc.
213 Danbury Road
Wilton, CT 06897
International: (203) 761-0042
Toll-free USA: (877) 226-8973
Fax: (203) 761-0043
www.4yourtype.com

www.dadamo.com—For All Things Peter D'Adamo

One of the longest running websites on the Internet, www.dadamo.com is the home page for the community of netizens who follow the work of Dr. Peter D'Adamo. This easy-to-navigate site is chockful of helpful tools, blogs, and one of the warmest, most welcoming chat forums to be found. Newbies are welcome to this moderated, family-friendly community.

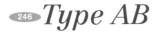

Dr. D'Adamo's products used in this book and where to find them:

Protein Blend™ Powder—Type B/AB

Dr. D'Adamo created a specific protein powder to benefit the individual needs of each blood type. The Type AB powder has a high protein content based on whole whey concentrate, and contains no sugar.

Protein Blend™ Powder can be purchased online at www.4yourtype .com. Simply click "Specialty Products" and scroll down to "Bars and Shakes."

Unibar® Protein Bar

The Unibar® is the healthy snack you don't have to feel guilty about! Designed by Dr. D'Adamo for all blood types, including Secretors and Non-Secretors, the Unibar® is ideal as a meal replacement, clean-fuel workout bar, or nutritious snack for a burst of energy between meals.

Chocolate Cherry (15 grams of protein) and Blueberry Almond (13 grams of protein) Unibar®s can be purchased online at www.4yourtype .com. Simply click "Specialty Products" and scroll down to "Bars and Shakes."

Carob Extract™

This delicious, irresistible syrup made from the carob bean is *Beneficial* for all blood types for easing digestive discomfort as well as coping with fatigue. It's so good that 1 teaspoon a day won't be enough! Use as a topping on crêpes, ice cream, muffins, and even cereals.

Carob Extract™ can be purchased online at www.4yourtype.com. Simply click "Specialty Products" and scroll down to find "Bars and Shakes."

Proberry 3™ Liquid

Developed for immune support, Proberry 3™ comes in both capsules and liquid . . . but after tasting the liquid you will be hooked! I drink it by the teaspoonful when I have a cold, or drizzle it in smoothies, mix in ice cream, or stir into tea for a tasty boost of antioxidants.

Proberry 3™ can be purchased online at www.4yourtype.com, simply click "Right for All Types" then "Immune Support," and scroll down to find Proberry 3™ Liquid.

For a complete list of all products formulated by Dr. Peter J. D'Adamo, go to www.4yourtype.com.

SWAMI© Personalized Nutrition Software Program

Dr. D'Adamo developed the SWAMI© software to harness the power of computers and artificial intelligence, using their tremendous precision and speed to help tailor unique one-of-a kind diets.

From its extensive knowledge base, SWAMI© can evaluate more than 700 foods for more than 200 individual attributes (such as cholesterol level, gluten content, presence of antioxidants, etc.) to determine if that food is either a superfood or toxin for you. It provides a specific one-of-a-kind diet in an easy-to-read, friendly format. For more information about SWAMI©, you can go to www.4yourtype.com.

References

1. Bob's Red Mill. Bob's Red Mill Natural Foods. www.bobsredmill.com. Accessed May 2013.

2. D'Adamo, Peter J., and Whitney, Catherine. *Eat Right 4 Your Blood Type.* New York: G. P. Putnam's Sons, 1996.

3. D'Adamo, Peter J., and Whitney, Catherine. *Live Right 4 Your Blood Type.* New York: G. P. Putnam's Sons, 2001.

4. "EWG's Shopper's Guide to Pesticides in Produce." Environmental Working Group, www.ewg.org, 2011.

5. "Food Labeling/Organic Foods." United States Department of Agriculture, www.usda.gov. Accessed May 2013.

6. Healthy Child, Healthy World. October 23, 2011. www.healthychild.org.

7. Mateljan, George. "The World's Healthiest Foods," www.whfoods.com. Accessed May 2013.

8. Nischan, Michel, and Goodbody, Mary. *Sustainably Delicious: Making the World a Better Place, One Recipe at a Time.* New York: Rodale Books, 2010.

Acknowledgments

PETER J. D'ADAMO

It is with great pleasure to share with the readers of *Eat Right 4 Your Type* and followers of my work on the Blood Type Diet® and my continuing explorations in the area of personalized medicine the *Eat Right 4 Your Type Personalized Cookbook* series. There are many people I would like to thank, as this was a group effort.

My deep appreciation to Berkley Books, a division of Penguin Group (USA), as my longtime publisher; in particular, my editor, Denise Silvestro, whose personal belief in these cookbooks brought them from their original e-book format to where we are today; publisher, Leslie Gelbman; Allison Janice, who coordinated the production efforts; Pam Barricklow, the managing editor; and the entire Berkley team who worked on these books. I would also like to thank my dedicated agent, Janis Vallely, whose encouragement, guidance, and tenacity have made this book possible.

A very special thanks to Kristin O'Connor, whose culinary skills, combined with her depth of knowledge of and belief in the Blood Type Diet®, have allowed us to develop delicious, nutritious recipes that are right for each type.

A special nod of appreciation for our team at North American Pharmacal and Drum Hill, who worked on these books as they were being developed, especially Bob Messineo, Wendy Simmons-Taylor, Ann Quasarano, John Alvord, Emily D'Adamo, and Angela Bergamini.

As always, I am grateful to my wife and partner, Martha Mosko D'Adamo, for her unwavering support and for the role she played in shepherding these books into existence; and to my two daughters, Claudia and Emily, who share a deep passion for this work and for a well-cooked meal.

A final thanks to the hundreds of thousands of readers and followers who have shared this journey with me. I am encouraged and fortified by your continuing dedication to your personal health and well-being, and I am humbled by your trust and commitment to this work.

KRISTIN O'CONNOR

I am so fortunate to have such a huge arena of support; I truly could not have done it without any of you.

First, of course is Dr. Peter D'Adamo, the science behind this effective diet. I will always respect your brilliant mind and interest in making this world a healthier place. To my mother, Susan O'Connor, for being the reason I had so much faith in this diet, teaching me how to cook, supporting my every move, and being there by my side while I tested all six hundred recipes! To my father, Kevin O'Connor, who sees more potential in me than anyone I've ever met, guided me in the basics of photography, and taught me to have the courage to put myself out there over and over again. To my brother, Dr. Ryan O'Connor, for valuing my accomplishments and always sharing in the joy of my success as if it were his own . . . and being a very willing recipe-testing guinea pig! To my grandparents Mike and Ellie DeMaio, thank you for being my cheerleaders, and for providing encouragement and unconditional support.

A huge thank you to David Domedion for utilizing his expertise to meticulously edit every recipe. Thank you to Chris Bierlein for his incredible talent, kind spirit, and generosity with shooting and editing our gorgeous cover photos. We were privileged to work with both of you.

Heather Rahilly, whose friendship kept me sane and whose intellect kept me in the race, thank you for being the most thorough attorney I could ask for! To my friends, who are all like family to me, for selflessly offering help in any way they could: Annie Gaffron, Mandy Geisler, Latha Chirunomula (along with Padma and Pushpavathi, for teaching me the basics of South Indian cooking), Jennifer Eastes, Iwona Lacka, and the Metwallys.

Thank you to Tim Macklin for being my very patient mentor, a great source of knowledge, and encouragement. Thanks to Danielle Boccher, Scott Olnhausen, and the rest of my pals at Concentric! Special thanks to Dr. Peter Bongiorno and Dr. Pina LoGiudice for taking me under their wing when I was just a little fledgling cook wanting to make a difference.

Thank you to Kate Fitzpatrick and Ann Quasarano, whose dependability and efforts at getting our book out there in the public eye was very much appreciated. Thanks to Stephen Czick for his hours of editing and support, and Wendy Simmons-Taylor for all her patience with styling these books.

Thanks to Martha D'Adamo and the team at Drum Hill Publishing for giving me the opportunity to work on these cookbooks that I very much love and believe in.

And finally, a very special thank you to Craig Anderson for taking a chance on me at the very beginning and opening the doors to my dreams.

PETER J. D'ADAMO

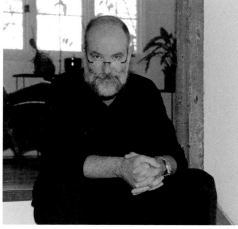

Photo credit: Susan Morrow

A second-generation naturopathic doctor, Dr. D'Adamo has been practicing naturopathic medicine for more than thirty years. Best known for his research on human blood groups and nutrition, Dr. D'Adamo is also a well-respected researcher in the field of natural products and a Distinguished Professor of Clinical Sciences at the University of Bridgeport. He is the founder and director of the Center of Excellence in Generative Medicine, a clinical, academic, and research institute, which also houses his private clinical practice located in a beautifully restored Victorian house on the campus of the University of Bridgeport overlooking the Long Island Sound. Dr. D'Adamo is the recipient of the 1990 AANP Physician of the Year Award for his role in the creation of the *Journal of Naturopathic Medicine*. Dr. D'Adamo's series of books are *New York Times* bestsellers and Book-of-the-Month Club selections. He was named the "Most Intriguing Health Author of 1999," and his first book, *Eat Right 4 Your Type*, was voted one of the "Ten Most Influential Health Books of All Time" by media industry analysts. *Publishers Weekly* called his third book, *Live Right 4 Your Type*, "A comprehensive and fascinating theory that has been meticulously researched." His books have been translated into sixty-five languages, and there are over 7 million copies of his books worldwide.

KRISTIN O'CONNOR

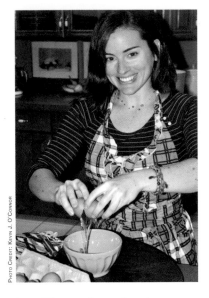

Photo Credit: Kevin J. O'Connor

Kristin O'Connor has made it her life's work to create food that is irresistibly tasty and healthy, a combination she hopes will inspire people to love good, healthy food and encourage them to make it a lifelong habit. In doing so, she created NourishThis.com—a website with recipes, articles, and tips on eating well and living green; volunteers for Healthy Child, Healthy World—a non-profit that educates parents about nutritional and environmental issues affecting their children; and presented at the Kids Food Festival in New York City. She has worked for a Food Network and Cooking Channel production company as an associate producer on many of their shows, was an above-the-line catering chef for a lead actor on a major motion picture, and is now working as a private celebrity chef. Kristin continues to volunteer for nonprofit organizations that promote a healthy diet and environment, and hopes to continue her career as a cookbook author in the future.

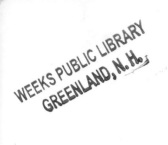